THE
RAINBOW
DIET

THE RAINBOW DIET

A Holistic Approach to Radiant Health
through Foods and Supplements

DEANNA MINICH, PHD

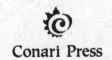

Conari Press

This edition first published in 2018 by Conari Press, an imprint of

Red Wheel/Weiser, LLC
With offices at:
65 Parker Street, Suite 7
Newburyport, MA 01950
www.redwheelweiser.com

ISBN: 978-1-57324-687-3

Library of Congress Cataloging-in-Publication Data

Names: Minich, Deanna, author.
Title: The rainbow diet : unlock the ancient secrets to health through foods
    and supplements / Deanna M. Minich, PhD.
Description: Newburyport, MA : Conari Press, 2018. | Includes bibliographical
    references.
Identifiers: LCCN 2016032445 | ISBN 9781573246873 (paperback)
Subjects: LCSH: Nutrition--Popular works. | Self-care, Health--Popular works.
    | BISAC: HEALTH & FITNESS / Diets. | HEALTH & FITNESS / Nutrition.
Classification: LCC RA784 .M5152 2018 | DDC 613.2--dc23
LC record available at https://lccn.loc.gov/2016032445

Cover design by Jim Warner
Cover illustration © Linda Vostrovska / shutterstock
Interior by Deborah Dutton
Typeset in Adobe Garamond Pro and Gotham
Printed in Canada
MAR

10 9 8 7 6 5 4 3 2 1

TO RAINBOWS AND ALL RAINBOW WARRIORS

When the Earth is ravaged and the animals are dying, a new tribe of people shall come unto the Earth from many colors, creeds, and classes, and who by their actions and deeds shall make the earth green again. They shall be known as the Warriors of the Rainbow.

Hopi prophecy

TABLE OF CONTENTS

NOTE TO READERS

This book contains advice and information relating to health and is not meant to diagnose, treat, or prescribe. It should be used to supplement, rather than replace, the advice of your physician or other trained healthcare practitioner. If you know or suspect you have a medical condition, are experiencing physical symptoms, or if you feel unwell, I recommend that you seek your physician's advice before embarking on any health program or treatment.

Every effort possible was made to ensure the accuracy of the information contained in this book as of the date of its publication. Since the research on food and dietary supplements is ever-changing, however, new developments will undoubtedly be revealed over time. It is the responsibility of individual readers to consult with experts and current literature for future updates on foods, vitamins, minerals, and supplements that may be relevant to their physical conditions, including changes in dosage, duration of use, side effects, or for treating or preventing conditions.

In addition, please note that this book is not a comprehensive guide to all foods and supplements that exist for all conditions. Only a select group of supplements is included. For any medical condition or symptom, always consult with a qualified physician or appropriate healthcare professional. Neither the author nor the publisher accepts any responsibility for your health, how you choose to use the information contained in this book, or your medical outcomes resulting from applying the methods suggested in this book. Names and identifying details have been changed to honor individuals' desire for confidentiality.

INTRODUCTION

We are indeed much more than what we eat, but what we eat can nevertheless help us to be much more than what we are.

Adelle Davis

When I was a pre-teen, my mother experienced an inner revelation about food and faith. She became conscious of what she ate and what she believed. At the time I was witnessing her metamorphosis, I wasn't too thrilled. My life as a sugar-loving child changed radically, as I could no longer have unhealthy, processed foods and eat candy as my peers did. By the age of nine, I had learned how to read food labels, and I was bringing wholesome food to school for lunch. At the time, I didn't realize the value in having this leg up on my health or the value of changing my mindset about eating.

My teenage years were filled with emotional tumult about food. I became a secret sugar addict, binging on cookies, candy, cake, and anything I could sneak away from home. I overate, ate for emotional reasons, and ate in response to stress. My skin broke out, my hormones were all over the place, and I developed rather severe premenstrual syndrome (PMS) and endometriosis. Aside from what was happening to my body, I was moody and emotional, and instead of confronting these emotions, I turned to food for comfort.

In school, I always had a fascination with the human body. Human biology was my favorite subject, and I spent hours in the library reading anatomy and physiology textbooks. By the age of eighteen, I had a subscription to the *Journal of the American Medical Association*, a top-tier medical journal. I was all set to be a medical doctor and surely had no interest in nutrition. I went to college and chose pre-med as my major, with a focus on biology.

My gut, skin, and reproductive organs continued to give me problems during my studies. In addition to researching the body in my science classes, I began searching in other places for answers to my health problems. I signed up for a yoga class because I had heard from others how it helped them. The class opened me up to a new world of thinking and movement in my body. I can still remember the revelation vividly even now. I was so enthused that I decided to explore further.

I began signing up for classes that were not my usual "type." Philosophy, religion, and literature courses began to fill my semester schedules as I became increasingly intrigued by these decidedly non-medical subjects.

I worked during the summer as temporary help at doctors' offices, including an ophthalmologist, an internist, and two different cardiologists. I spent one summer as a volunteer at a hospital. Each summer that passed, however, brought more and more doubts about going to medical school. I didn't like the way I saw patients moving through their visits—not really getting the answers to *why* they had certain conditions. They were only provided with pharmaceutical and surgical solutions to their problems. I just couldn't put my heart into it. Medicine felt like an all-or-nothing profession to me, and I wasn't seeing it as my "all." I began noticing that it wasn't just pills, but also food and lifestyle, that made a difference in a person's health. I also noticed some personal health changes as I moved away from eating sugary foods and started eating more vegetables and whole foods.

Finally, in my junior year in college, when I needed to take the MCAT to get into medical school, I had an inner epiphany: *This is not my path*. I did what I had never thought I would do: I signed up for graduate school to study nutrition science. I felt that I wanted to do something to prevent medical symptoms rather than commit my life to just treating them. Maybe my mother was right all along!

I chose to study nutrition science during a three-year master's degree and then completed a four-year program for my PhD. While I focused on nutritional research in my professional life, in my personal life I was on a parallel track studying other forms of healing truths—Ayurveda, Traditional Chinese Medicine (TCM), herbal medicine, functional medicine, and some more "alternative" forms of nutrition that I wasn't taught in graduate school.

I soon discovered that ancient healing traditions and modern science were all interconnected. Many of the ancient secrets held within Asian healing traditions were now being validated by science through research.

I was particularly interested in the ancient "pivot points" in the body where a lot of activity happens. These spots are aligned to the endocrine system we know in physiology—the adrenal glands, the ovaries (in women) and testes (in men), the pancreas, the heart and thymus, and the thyroid, pituitary, and pineal glands. My preoccupation with hormones and the endocrine system grew to encompass the larger physiological functions of these glands integrated with their symbolic role in ancient traditions like Ayurveda and yoga. What drew me even more was the association of these seven endocrine glands to colors, a connection well-established in the older healing traditions. My study of the colorful carotenoids and phytonutrients in graduate school had shown me that there is an important "color connection" in nutrition science, and now I was seeing it in the long-recognized system of endocrine organs.

I began to realize that color, nutrition, and life issues were intertwined, and when I began my clinical practice over fifteen years ago, I started to see these correlations rather distinctly.

As a scientist and questioning truth-seeker, I put together the Rainbow Diet, which brings together the full spectrum of a person's health. I've been using the Rainbow Diet as a system to help people for years, and have found it to be an eye-opening experience. Unlike most traditional restrictive "diets," the Rainbow Diet is about finding the foods, supplements, and eating styles that fit your unique, personal physiology and psychology. As a clinical and research-oriented nutritionist, I've never believed in the "one-diet-fits-all" approach. It just didn't seem realistic based on what I had learned about individual biochemistry and genetic variability.

Quite simply, the Rainbow Diet, is an organizing framework to put your body, psychology, eating, and living together into one view. This is important, because many nutrition paradigms or diets are fragmented. They see the foods you eat, but not your lifestyle and how everything is interconnected. The Rainbow Diet provides a real-time navigation map that gets you where you need to be with food, taking into consideration all aspects of your life. I'll use the colors of the rainbow to help guide you through:

- Red for the grounding, physical issues of your body
- Orange for your creative, playful, emotional side
- Yellow for the bright radiance of your intellect
- Green for the expansion of your heart
- Aquamarine to represent your personal truths and speaking
- Indigo for the deeper knowledge and intuition we all carry
- White for your spiritual self, or your ability to be connected with something greater

In this book, you will learn not just about how to eat a rainbow diet, but also how to live a rainbow life that is a perfect fit for you. In the first chapter, I show you how your life can be changed by following this path. I tell you about people who have embraced the Rainbow Diet and what their results have been. You will have the opportunity to take a Spectrum Quiz to see if you are living the rainbow life. After you know your scores, I recommend that you read each of the seven chapters that follow so you can see what each color means for you. You can read about how each color looks in your life and whether it is balanced. I show you ways to help balance your life, and recommend foods and supplements that can help. Then I help you put it all together to make sense in your life through an easy seven-day program to get you on track.

Ready to get your rainbow on? Let's go!

HOW TO USE THIS BOOK

I recommend that you read the first couple of chapters so you understand the general framework of the Rainbow Diet. Next, take the Spectrum Quiz so you can understand more about yourself and how you can maximize your results from the Rainbow Diet. Then go through the chapters that are most relevant to you, based on your scores. I also suggest keeping this book as a reference and a guide for foods and supplements that are tailored to your health issues.

CHAPTER 1

WHAT IS THE RAINBOW DIET?

Whole life is a search for beauty. But, when the beauty is found inside, the search ends and a beautiful journey begins.

Harshit Walia

We all contain the rainbow within. The Rainbow Diet will help you make sure that all your colors are shining brightly and in balance with each other. Before you take the Spectrum Quiz to find out about your rainbow, let me first describe to you each of the colors and what they represent. Each color has an overall meaning, as well as specific relationships to your body, nutrition, and life issues.

Red/ROOT

The color red represents the physical body and the boundaries you experience within the physical world in which you live. It also relates to feeling safe and secure in your identity. I call it the ROOT, because it is the anchor or "root" of your physical existence.

The ROOT gives you physical form and includes the following organs and systems:

Adrenal glands
Blood
Bones
DNA (your ancestral identity)
Feet
Immune system

Joints

Legs

Muscles

Rectum

Skin

Tailbone

It controls specific physiological activities:

Enzyme action

Excretion of substances that we do not need (e.g., feces)

Fight-or-flight response

Genomic expression

Protein production

As you will learn in the chapters to come, the ROOT is associated with foods and supplements that add to the structure and defenses of the body, for example:

Dietary protein

Immune-enhancing foods like medicinal mushrooms

Insoluble fiber to help with elimination

Mineral-rich foods to fortify the skeleton

Red-colored foods that are high in vitamin C

Root vegetables

The ROOT relates to important life issues as well, including:

Community/tribe

Safety

Survival

A Healthy Red/ROOT

People who are comfortable with their physical selves know that they can survive adequately in the world. They are able to receive from or provide support to a family or tribe. They are trustworthy and trust others. They accept themselves, especially their physical bodies and their earthly existence. They maintain healthy boundaries and believe they have a right to exist.

An Unhealthy Red/ROOT

People who are uncomfortable with their physical selves are less able to accomplish these things. Here are some indications that your red/ROOT may need some help.

Do you feel at odds with your family of origin?

People with ROOT imbalances usually struggle with physical-world issues, especially things like acquiring a home or shelter, making a living, or carrying on family traditions. These individuals often find it difficult to bond with family members in a way that is meaningful and solidifies a feeling of unity and cohesion.

Do you expend internal resources to feel safe?

When you are preoccupied with the stress of continually being on guard, you may ultimately tap into the inner adrenal and immune reserves you need to protect yourself from physical invaders like micro-organisms, viruses, excess inflammatory compounds, and toxins. Lower internal (immune) defenses may eventually lead to symptoms of bodily fatigue, frequent cold or flu, or inflammatory or autoimmune conditions.

Do you struggle with your daily survival?

Those with a ROOT imbalance may feel everyday life is difficult and not worth the effort. They can lack motivation and appear lazy to others, and may enter a deep depression. As a result, they can appear spacey, flighty, or not present. In fact, it may seem that they are not really "in their bodies." Without being fully present, you will have trouble living life fully and manifesting your dreams into physical reality.

Larry: No Boundaries

Larry has poor boundaries with others. He can easily start to take on other people's behaviors and emotions. When he sees someone crying, his eyes well up with tears. If someone is angry, he feels rage swelling from within. As a result, Larry finds himself confused around others. As a taxi driver who is around a wide variety of people, he often comes home at the end of the day feeling "spaced out." Many times, his body collapses in fatigue; he gets colds easily. He spends most of his free time in isolation so his life feels less complicated, which only adds to the problem of not having supportive social networks to engage him. Larry forgets to eat and, when he does, finds he is eating the same things over and over. He thinks he should avoid certain foods because he gets joint pain after eating them.

It is clear that Larry has an imbalance in his red/ROOT. He is not rooted in his own identity and doesn't have good boundaries to keep him feeling safe and secure in his core. He also seems to be losing his energy to others and through his food choices.

Orange/FLOW

The color orange represents your emotions and creativity. It is referred to as the FLOW, mainly because emotions are meant to do just that—be flowing and in motion!

The FLOW parts of us are fluid and flowing, including:

Bladder
Hips
Kidneys
Large intestine (colon)
Reproductive system
Sacrum

The FLOW oversees these physiological activities:

Cell growth
Fat storage
Reproduction
Water balance

The FLOW is associated with foods and supplements that encourage fluidity in the body, including:

Dietary fats and oils
Fermented foods
Fish and seafood
Nuts and seeds
Orange-colored foods
Tropical foods
Water

The FLOW regulates these life issues:

Creativity
Emotions
Relationships

A Healthy Orange/FLOW

Those who are comfortable with their emotional, creative selves can tap into their creative potential. They are comfortable expressing emotions. They "go with the flow" of life and live their life's dreams. They maintain healthy relationships with others, yet honor their own uniqueness. They have fun by engaging in pleasurable activities.

An Unhealthy Orange/FLOW

Here are some indications that your orange/FLOW may need some motion.

Do you feel unable to express emotions and creativity?

A sure sign of a FLOW imbalance is feeling "stuck" or stagnant and unable to move to action in your life. When your FLOW is blocked, you can't create or emote. You tend to be more prone to emotional eating, since you do not *feel* your feelings—you literally stuff them down with foods and constant eating. Your body may tend to be either too swollen or too dehydrated, indicating an impairment in the control of bodily fluids.

Do you feel unsatisfied in your relationships with others?

Have you been in relationships that are not equal, or that contain a degree of uncertainty or instability? Do you allow yourself to be abused emotionally? Is commitment to a relationship or a creative project an ongoing struggle? Follow-through is often difficult for individuals who aren't "flowing." Typically, they are good at coming up with ideas or starting a relationship, living in the high of the initial creative burst or romantic flair, but they find that things soon fail. They succumb to the eventual "I am not a creative person" or "I'd rather be alone"—which leaves them unable to come full circle with any aspect of life other than the repetition of this debilitating pattern.

Do you experience dysfunction in your sexuality?

Medical issues with your reproductive organs (for example, your uterus, ovaries, or testes) may indicate a problem with your FLOW. Imbalanced FLOW may also appear as meaningless sexual encounters, or as abstinence and fear concerning sexuality, stemming from experience or from family patterns that have been passed on.

Sasha: All Sparkle, No Substance

Sasha adorns herself with bright, colorful clothes. She thrives on the drama occurring at the retail store she works in and fills her spare time watching entertainment channels to find out the latest in Hollywood. Her friends see her as a creative person who is in a state of constant emotional flux. On the surface, Sasha appears extremely friendly, making conversation with everyone she meets. She involves herself in a number of relationships, although she is unable to commit to any of them fully. As a result, intimate connections start out very intensely for Sasha, but are often ended by her because of her inability to commit emotionally. Finally, Sasha has a history of recurring ovarian cysts. Her diet is filled with processed foods, which she relies on for comfort when she is feeling emotional.

Sasha is topsy-turvy in her orange FLOW. She is highly emotional, but hasn't found a way to express herself so that she feels balanced in relationships. Her rollercoaster moods lead her to emotional eating and food cravings.

Yellow/FIRE

The color yellow stands for the bright radiance of your thinking self and the energy that fuels your busy world of activities. It is referred to as the FIRE, since it connects to how we harness our energy and transform our lives, whether it's our thoughts or food.

The FIRE in your body sparks those parts that relate to energy and transformation, including:

Gallbladder
Liver
Pancreas
Small intestine
Stomach

It organizes these physiological activities:

Assimilation of nutrients from food
Blood-sugar balance
Digestion
Transformation of food into energy

The FIRE is associated with foods and supplements that assist with transformation and energy balance, including:

Dietary carbohydrates
Healthy sweeteners
Legumes
Soluble fiber (including those found in moist fruits, psyllium, and
    flaxseed meal)
Whole grains (gluten-free preferred for those with intolerance or
    allergy)
Yellow-colored foods

The FIRE regulates these life issues:

Balance
Energy
Power

A Healthy Yellow/FIRE

Those who sit within their powerful, fiery selves keep their work/life balance. They wield their personal power in the world and transform thoughts from the outer world with internal beliefs and opinions. They think logically and and use their life experiences to give them energy.

An Unhealthy Yellow/FIRE

Here are some indications that your yellow/FIRE may need either rekindling or healing from burnout.

Do you feel stressed by the responsibilities of life?

Do situations, no matter how small or large, seem to tax your internal reserves? Is your life drained of any "sweetness" and beset by burdens? Are you tired all the time? Do you remain unsatisfied from eating? When your inner FIRE is "burnt out," there is a drain on your entire being, preventing it from interacting with the outside world in ways that are nourishing. Mental stress or fatigue typically result. Eating becomes erratic and your appetite may become insatiable due to a lack of fulfillment from daily experience. Life feels like drudgery when you are without FIRE energy.

Are you overweight, particularly in the abdomen?

Do you suffer from digestive complaints like indigestion, acid reflux, or bloating? When there is excessive, unprocessed fuel in your digestive tract and in your body overall, it may result in too much belly fat, too much acid, too much gas, and/or too much undigested food.

Do you lack self-confidence, or are you egotistical?

Do you analyze your achievements to the extent that you discount them or inflate them out of proportion? Are you a perfectionist or obsessive with details? Are you driven to the point of excess, trying to "do it all," believing that you can do everything on your own? The FIRE is an action-oriented aspect, but sometimes ambition and motivation shift into high gear and go on auto-pilot or into overdrive. These states are clearly unhealthy and unbalanced. They can ultimately lead to exhaustion and the "never enough" syndrome, in which no object, event, or accomplishment is satisfying.

Tom: On the Brink of Burnout

Tom has a "can-do" attitude. He became the CEO of his startup company at age twenty-five, and a self-made multi-millionaire by the age of forty-two. His nature is to forge through situations fiercely and competitively, with an edge of anger, often leaving others emotionally bruised and battered in his wake. The people who work for him find him inspiring at times, but mostly overbearing and self-righteous.

Tom lives a fast life, eating on the run between meetings or during travel—if he remembers to eat at all. His digestion has progressively worsened, and he experiences belching and acid in his stomach after eating. These symptoms do not stop him from pursuing his incessant activity, and he continues to push himself to do more. Lately, he has found himself oversleeping on the weekends, feeling so fatigued that he cannot push himself out of bed. However, he still pushes himself in order to keep his business profitable. Throughout the years, Tom's weight has been increasing and, recently, his doctor told him that his cholesterol is high and that he is heading in the direction of becoming diabetic.

From the outside, you could say that Tom's FIRE is burning bright. He appears to be a successful man in that he has wielded his power to become financially secure and own his own business. Although Tom may be the CEO, however, he is not a leader in his core. Rather, he operates from a place of inflated self-esteem and ego so that he can mask the insecurity he feels about his self and abilities. He uses force and competition as a means to get what he wants. His addiction to keeping busy prevents him from looking at the real issues in his life that need evaluation. Instead, he busies his mind with excessive analytical and logical thoughts ("analysis paralysis"), squashing his inherent intuitive sense.

Through the excess acid and fatigue that he feels, Tom's body has been signaling to him that he is in overdrive and needs to slow down. Tom ignores these signals, denying that there is a problem. This is symbolic of his belief that he is ultimately "calling the shots." His greatest healing would involve removing old thought patterns so that he can move confidently in the direction that promotes the highest good for him and others.

Green/LOVE

The color green represents the healing qualities of love. It is referred to as the LOVE, signifying our compassion and devotion to ourselves and others.

The LOVE in your body nourishes systems of expansion, opening, and giving. These include:

Armpits
Arms
Blood vessels
Breasts
Hands
Heart
Lungs
Lymphatic system
Shoulders
Wrists

The LOVE is connected to these physiological activities:

Breathing
Circulation
Oxygenation

The LOVE is associated with foods and supplements rich in nutrients that open up the circulation and increase oxygenation, for example:

Leafy vegetables (e.g., salad greens)
Microgreens
Phytonutrients and plant foods
Sprouts
Vegetables

The LOVE regulates these life issues:

Compassion
Expansion
Healing

A Healthy Green/LOVE

Those who are nurtured by their loving selves express love, give thanks, and are grateful. They embrace love as the underlying foundation for everything they do. They love themselves and others, and are able to give and receive in equal measure.

An Unhealthy Green/LOVE

Here are some indications that your green/LOVE may need some caretaking.

Do you over-give to or over-receive from others?

Do you feel it is difficult to say "no" to others and are you resentful when you don't say "no"? Does over-nurturing lead you to feel exhausted and bitter? Keeping the LOVE in balance by having a healthy mix of receiving and giving is essential. Over-giving is often encouraged in modern society, but it can deplete your heart in the long-term. Giving the LOVE inside you permission to receive can be liberating. And in the end, it can allow you to be better at giving to others.

Do you suffer from heart or breathing difficulties?

Do you have difficulty eating healthily or taking care of yourself? Constriction and lack of energy flow in the heart area can contribute to heart and circulatory problems. Heart disease is the number-one killer in most industrialized societies. What is causing this restriction and pain in the heart? Stress, lack of passion, or lack of love may all be contributing to the heart-disease epidemic.

Has your heart suffered deep, emotional trauma?

Have you had emotional wounds that have impaired your ability to give and receive love? Wounds that cannot be resolved? Are you unable to forgive others? A wounded heart can lead to a belief that life is full of sadness and grief. Being closed off from your deepest feelings results in a numb feeling about life. Those with a LOVE imbalance may not be able to cry or to touch and be touched by others.

Melanie: A Loss of Heart

At the age of six, Melanie lost her father to pancreatic cancer. It was a trag-ic, quick death that left Melanie reeling with mixed emotions. Her mother was grief-stricken and not able to give Melanie the comfort or attention that she needed at the time. Instead, she chose to ignore her hurt and to enter into a new relationship with an abusive man. Melanie was frightened by her mother's new lover and spent much time tucked away in her small bedroom on her own. In the years that followed, Melanie became more of a loner, spending time away from home whenever possible. She found ways to keep herself busy and distracted, usually by staying late after school and by losing herself in fiction at the local library.

As an adult, Melanie found herself unable truly to love others, even in intimate relationships. Her heart remained stifled and stagnant. In her for-ties, she developed breathing difficulties that eventually turned into asth-ma. At her core, Melanie lost sight of what it meant to feel. She was only able to tap into the loneliness and isolation she had felt for most of her life since her father's death.

Melanie displays an imbalanced LOVE. Her whole life is a woven thread of grief and sorrow. This trauma remains lodged somewhere in the caverns of her heart rather than being expressed. These trapped feelings strongly impact her ability to give and receive love.

Aquamarine/TRUTH

The color aquamarine signifies truth-telling and truth-speaking. I have simply called it the TRUTH, but it carries the complexity of being true to yourself as well as the verbal expression of your personal truths.

The TRUTH in your body connects to systems that allow for verbal expression, including:

Cheeks
Chin
Ears
Mouth
Neck
Nose

Throat

Thyroid gland

It is linked to these physiological activities:

Chewing

Hearing

Metabolism

Smelling

Speaking

Foods and supplements for the TRUTH are those that lubricate and open channels of expression, including:

Fruits

Juice

Sauces

Sea plants

Soups and stews

Teas

Life issues regulated by the TRUTH include:

Authenticity

Choice

Voice

A Healthy Aquamarine/TRUTH

Those who express their TRUTH speak their truths. They express themselves through their voice and open up to who they authentically are. They approach choices and make decisions with confidence.

An Unhealthy Aquamarine/TRUTH

Here are some indications that your aquamarine/TRUTH may need some expression.

Do you feel inhibited or overly open when communicating?

Your voice is a conduit for personal expression and creativity. Do you have a tendency to talk too much, trying to fill the silence or dodge important issues related to communication? Or are you silent because of a lack of connection with your stream of creativity? How you use your voice says volumes about the health of your TRUTH. When your TRUTH is imbalanced, it may shut down, resulting in a suffocating feeling. Or it may become too excessive and open, to the extent that nothing gets held back. Words can become as sharp as razors, or be turned into garbled nonsense. If you are cut off from your wellspring of creativity, your TRUTH will become desiccated and your voice raspy.

Are you avoiding your authentic self?

Those with TRUTH imbalance may shy away from their personal values and inner truths, and deny who they really are. They may fear the consequences of exposing themselves, because it might mean criticism, judgment, or exclusion. The more you can step into your true "blue" self, the more freedom you will feel, and the less you will be held back by the shackles of other people's opinions and perspectives.

Do you make choices that are consistent with your inner truth?

We vocalize our choices. When you speak your decisions from a place of hurry, lack, or excess, however, you are not in alignment with your TRUTH. You may also hold back on making the best decision for yourself because you don't want to be wrong or feel as if you are hurting others in the process. When you know your truths deep inside, you can let them be the guideposts to your decision-making and daily choices.

Bill: Nothing but Noise

Bill was asked by his manager to conduct computer training classes with large audiences. Upon hearing this news, Bill felt an uneasy tickling feeling in his throat, as there is a part of him that does not feel comfortable speaking in front of others. He doesn't want to fail, but knows that he also does not want to turn down the opportunity to please his boss.

Throughout his life, Bill has struggled with these and other choices, small and large. He has not been able to locate his "inner voice." Often, he looks outside of himself for validation and to help him arrive at a decision. Periodically, he reflects back to uncover decisions that he regrets, and has difficulty forgetting and moving on from them. His indecisiveness haunts him occasionally.

One of the reservations Bill has about public speaking is that he has some degree of speech difficulty. He notes that he inadvertently mixes words together. Also, when he was a child, his mother had him take speech therapy, and Bill felt ashamed for being unable to communicate effectively. Bill speaks rapidly and sometimes mumbles and rambles on in the presence of others simply to fill the space. Similarly, he eats to fill his time, even when he is not hungry. He feels uncomfortable with silence when with others, and also when he is alone. If at home by himself, he surrounds himself with the sounds of the television or radio. He quickly gulps his food, not paying attention to what he is eating. He has a lingering memory of almost choking to death when he was four years old.

Bill has a number of issues with his TRUTH. The most obvious ones are those related to his ability to communicate. Speaking has not always been fluid for him. Bill's TRUTH is on overdrive with his fast talking and mixing-up of words. A part of him is unwilling to take in sensory input; instead, he blocks it by talking excessively. On a deeper level, there may be things he does not want to hear.

Indigo/INSIGHT

The color indigo symbolizes the inner wisdom and intuition we all carry. This deeply blue-purple hue is known as the INSIGHT, or the inner sight we have.

The INSIGHT in your body connects to systems that allow for the function of the mind, memory, imagination, and intuition. These include:

Brain
Eyebrows
Eyes
Forehead
Neurons

Neurotransmitters
Pituitary gland

It is associated with these physiological activities:

Mood balance
Sleep
Thought processing

Foods and supplements for the INSIGHT are those that influence the mind, mood, and brain, including:

Blue-purple foods
Caffeine
Cocoa
Fats and oils
Spices

Life issues regulated by the INSIGHT include:

Discernment
Reflection
Visualization

A Healthy Indigo/INSIGHT

People who are in tune with their intuitive selves follow their dreams. They process thoughts within a larger context of experience and separate wisdom from illusion. They understand the value of heeding intuition and have balanced moods.

An Unhealthy Indigo/INSIGHT

Here are some indications that your indigo/INSIGHT may need some focus.

Do your dreams sometimes seem more real than your waking life?
Do you have erratic sleep patterns, like consistently sleeping fewer than five hours or more than nine? Do you have vivid dreams that can some-

times be disturbing and real? An imbalanced INSIGHT reveals itself in changes in sleeping and dreaming. People who have haunting or extremely vivid dreams or who find themselves more intrigued with other realities than with the one in which they live may have excessive activity in their INSIGHT. Reining in this activity through supplements, dream journaling, and meditating can help to funnel intuitive activity better.

Do you tend to be overly analytical?

Do you constantly ruminate about your decisions or reactions to situations to the point of losing sight of the overall picture? Do you second-guess yourself? Are you obsessive-compulsive, trying to keep your thoughts in check and your surroundings suppressed? When thoughts get the better of you, your INSIGHT may need some cleaning out and reorganization. Wisdom needs to take the place of a nagging intellect.

Are you prone to depression or feeling cut off from reality?

Do you have difficulty staying in the present moment? Do you live more comfortably in your imagination or illusory life? Those with INSIGHT disturbances tend to seek ways to "get away from it all" by indulging in food or drink, particularly chocolate, coffee, or alcohol. They may use drugs or have used them in the past. An "addictive nature" represents the involvement of INSIGHT.

Tina: Spiraling into Another World

Tina finds herself waking up at night, plagued by nightmares. In the morning, she feels scattered and clumsy due to lack of sleep. Her friends describe her as a "complex" person, and her brother calls her "moody." He says that she is like a woman "who wears a thousand faces," because her disposition is always changing.

Although she is unable to spend much time with it, Tina feels best when she is expressing herself through art. When she doesn't paint, she feels like a different person. Her imagination takes over, causing her inner fantasy life to collide with her practical everyday life. As a result, she experiences chaos in her dealings with people and situations. She easily finds herself overwhelmed with life, and describes this as a "sensory overload."

Sometimes lights, noise, and color fill her mind and she is unable to function clearly.

Tina's INSIGHT is in high gear, giving her vivid dreams, an overactive imagination, and an uncontrollable flux of psychic activity. She becomes paralyzed by the influx of information coming in from both the outside and the inside. Individuals like Tina with INSIGHT complexity appear to be moody because they are responding to the stimuli they are constantly receiving.

White/SPIRIT

The color white connects to the spiritual self, which is why I use the word SPIRIT for this system. The spiritual self encompasses our sense of purpose and meaning, faith, and purification.

The SPIRIT is only subtly associated with the physical body. It is the fine wiring within, and includes:

Electromagnetic fields
Energy meridians
Nervous system
Pineal gland

It oversees these physiological activities:

Circadian rhythms
Cleansing and detoxification
Light sensitivity and receptivity

Since the SPIRIT is more about the spiritual self than the physical body, there are limited foods related to it. Here, we focus more on food withdrawal and cleansing:

Fasting
Foods that help with nervous-system function
Detoxifying foods
Photons (the role of light in food and nutrition)
Toxin-free foods

Life issues related to the SPIRIT include:

Connection
Meaning
Purpose/Calling

A Healthy White/SPIRIT

People who are comfortable with their spiritual, unified selves have faith in something greater than themselves. They pray or meditate for guidance and surrender their lives to their souls' calling. They integrate their earthly beings with their spirit selves and devote their lives to a greater purpose.

An Unhealthy White/SPIRIT

Here are some indications that your white/SPIRIT may require clarity and purity.

Are you preoccupied with your spirit?
Do you tend to live by such devout religious or spiritual tenets that you neglect your physical body to the extent that you have difficulty surviving? Do you neglect your physical body by not taking care of it (e.g., forgetting to eat, refusing to exercise, etc.)? A SPIRIT imbalance may result in a shift in priorities that may not benefit the whole self, just part of it. By not treating the body as a temple or a divine vehicle, you neglect part of you that is essential for living on this planet.

Do you lack intimate connection with something greater than yourself?
Do you feel deep despair over the purpose of living, or feel that "God has let you down"? Do you feel isolated? An imbalance in SPIRIT may result in a life that feels devoid of purpose due to the lack of interconnection with all physical and spiritual life.

Do you constantly question your spiritual existence?
On the other end of the spectrum, do you fail to see yourself as more than just your physical body? This kind of denial may also be a reflection of a stagnant SPIRIT. You may avoid a spiritual path because it may alter your life and you fear that you may not to able to accept the changes.

Keith: Closed to His Calling

Keith was raised in a very strict religious household. His mother, active in church affairs, required that Keith attend services every week with her. She also volunteered him for several church-related activities without his consent and donated much of the family money to the church, even though they didn't have much. As if that weren't enough, she earnestly expressed her wish that Keith become a pastor.

By the age of fifteen, Keith felt stifled by his mother's religiosity. At eighteen, he started to develop panic attacks. As a young adult, he withdrew from society by staying inside, and even stopped eating for days at a time. His panic attacks continued and he decided to get help from a psychiatrist. Medications appeared to work temporarily. Keith formed a close bond with a work colleague and told him about his panic attacks and family background. On a daily basis, he began unraveling the wounds of the past to allow enough room in his life to explore his own spirituality.

For Keith, his mother's approach to spirituality backfired. It polarized him and blocked him from any spiritual beliefs. With his blocked SPIRIT, he backed himself into a corner rather than connecting with the larger gift of life. This resulted in his panic attacks. The healing will occur when he can do his own soul-searching and find his own path of spirit.

CHAPTER 2

WHAT DOES YOUR INNER RAINBOW LOOK LIKE?

I kind of view everybody like a rainbow. Everybody on the planet has all the colors of the rainbow inside.

Alexia Fast

The easiest way for you to begin to understand the Rainbow Diet is for you to get to know your own colors and where you stand in your spectrum of health. I've developed the Spectrum Quiz so that you can see where you need to focus your attention. Allow about fifteen to twenty minutes to go through each question and answer as honestly as you can in the moment.

Of course, your responses may change depending on your circumstances. If you are stressed and at work, you may answer differently than if you are at home before bedtime feeling calm and relaxed. Try to take the quiz in your most natural, relaxed state, as your result will tell you where your optimal and maximal state of health resides. Take it again when you are feeling a bit more on edge in the midst of a busy day, as this will tell you where you have some vulnerability. I think it's important to see how your "colors" change when you move from one health state to another.

If you have to choose between the two situations—at work or at home—focus on where you have some room to improve. Taking the Spectrum Quiz after a busy day may be a good way to see where you stand when you are stressed. You can write out your scores on a piece of paper and then monitor them over time using the Spectrum Quiz Tracker in Appendix D.

The Spectrum Quiz

For each statement, answer either yes or no. When you are done, tally the number of "no" responses for each color. At the end of the quiz, I'll show you how to use your results going forward.

Red/ROOT

This section of the quiz assesses your body, food, and life issues as they relate to the color **red (ROOT)** and its connection to how you live in your **physical world**. It relates to themes of safety, survival, instinct, community, protein, and the body structures that provide strength and protection.

1. Do you feel good in your own skin?
2. Do you have good boundaries with others?
3. Do you feel safe in your body?
4. Do you feel safe in your home?
5. Are you free from any impending danger?
6. Do you find it easy to deal with daily stressors?
7. Do you work well under pressure?
8. Is surviving in your everyday world easy?
9. Do you go with your instincts?
10. Do you trust others?
11. Do you spend quality, nourishing time in your community?
12. Can you go to your community for help when you need it?
13. Are your social networks supportive?
14. Do you have family and/or close friends on whom you can rely?
15. Do you feel good about your family of origin and/or upbringing?
16. Do you take care of your body by eating regularly?
17. Do you eat protein throughout the day?
18. Do you avoid foods that disagree with you?
19. Do you eat natural, whole foods that are red in color—apples, cherries, etc.?

20. Does your body tend to feel better after eating?

21. Do you consider yourself to have a strong constitution?

22. Are you usually "the last one to get sick"?

23. Are you at a healthy body weight?

24. Is your skin clear?

25. Are you free of bone or joint pain and inflammation?

Orange/FLOW

This section of the quiz assesses your body, food, and life issues as they relate to the color **orange (FLOW)** and its connection to how you live in your **emotional world**. It deals with themes of emotional expression, creativity, playfulness, water, fats and oils, and the body structures that are creative and flowing.

1. Do you find it easy to express your emotions to others?

2. Do you readily "go with the flow" of how a situation is unfolding?

3. Do you express yourself when you feel something is "off"?

4. Are you able to move through your emotions so you don't overeat?

5. Are you generally in touch with your feelings?

6. Do you consider yourself creative?

7. Do you generally put your creative ideas into practical action?

8. Are you able to see possibilities in a situation that seems dismal?

9. Is your creativity nourished on a daily basis?

10. Do you enjoy being creative?

11. Do you make time for play?

12. Do you consider yourself playful?

13. Do you feel that you have enough fun in all you do?

14. Are you comfortable with your sexuality?

15. Are you able to create a healthy, nourishing partnership with another person?

16. Do you eat some healthy fats and oils every day?

17. Are you eating natural, whole foods that are orange in color (e.g., carrots, oranges)?

18. Do you eat foods that contain healthy oils (e.g., nuts, seeds, salmon)?

19. Do you think you drink enough water?

20. Do you drink fluids throughout the day?

21. Is your sex drive good?

22. Are your bowel movements of a normal consistency (no diarrhea or constipation)?

23. Do you feel adequately hydrated?

24. Do you engage in activities that make you sweat?

25. Are your hormones balanced?

Yellow/FIRE

This section of the quiz assesses your body, food, and life issues as they relate to the color **yellow (FIRE)** and its connection to how you live in your **thinking, busy world of activities**. It evaluates themes of energy level, thought patterns, ambition, work/life balance, carbohydrates, and digestion.

1. Do you have a good energy level compared to most people you know?

2. Do your daily activities give you energy?

3. Does being around people give you energy?

4. Do you feel energized and active after eating a meal?

5. Do you get a "high" when you accomplish projects or tasks?

6. Do you strive to do your best, yet not feel as if you have to do things perfectly?

7. Are you determined in your pursuits, yet keep your personal life balanced?

8. Are you focused on your goals, but also flexible if something comes up?

9. Are you more accepting of yourself rather than being self-critical?

10. Do you keep your ambitious goals in balance with enjoying life?

11. Do you maintain a healthy work/life balance?

12. Do you create opportunities for down time away from work?

13. Are you realistic about taking on work you can reasonably do without overcommitting?

14. Do you handle a busy schedule without fretting?

15. Do you only say "yes" to things you can comfortably do?

16. Do you avoid excessive sweets or desserts?

17. Do you avoid excessive amounts of starchy foods (e.g., breads, pastas, pretzels)?

18. Do you avoid quick-energy, caffeinated drinks?

19. Do you avoid sugary foods when you are stressed?

20. Do you cook more at home compared with eating out?

21. Would you say you have good digestion?

22. Do you have healthy blood-sugar levels?

23. Is your belly area trim?

24. Does your stomach feel comfortable after eating?

25. Do you feel as if your energy level is even throughout the day?

Green/LOVE

This section of the quiz assesses your body, food, and life issues as they relate to the color **green (LOVE)** and its connection to **love** in your life. It addresses self-love, compassion, devotion, green vegetables, the cardiovascular and respiratory systems, and circulation and oxygenation through physical activity.

1. Do you feel compassion for others?

2. Do you feel dedicated to a cause that you are connected to in your heart?

3. Are you quick to forgive and forget?

4. Are you a generous person and, at the same time, able to receive from others?

5. Are you able to be of service to others and, at the same time, let others help you?

6. Are you physically active?

7. Do you consider yourself physically fit?

8. Do you make time to be in nature?

9. Do you breathe deeply on a regular basis?

10. Do you do some aerobic activity on a regular basis—walking, biking, or running?

11. Do you make time for you?

12. Do you let others help you if you are in need?

13. Do you take care of yourself to the same extent you are able to take care of others?

14. Are you living out your heartfelt passions?

15. Do you make time to do what you love?

16. Do you eat plant-based foods every day?

17. Do you eat green vegetables (e.g., broccoli, kale, cabbage) at least three times per week?

18. Do you eat leafy green salads at least every other day?

19. Do you feel grateful for your daily meals?

20. Do you love eating vegetables of all types?

21. Are your hands and feet comfortably warm?

22. Can you breathe without difficulty?

23. Is it easy to breathe while you exercise?

24. Is your blood pressure normal?

25. Is your heart rate normal?

Aquamarine/TRUTH

This section of the quiz assesses your body, food, and life issues as they relate to the color **aquamarine (TRUTH)** and its connection to **truth-telling** in your life. It deals with being true to yourself, expressing yourself verbally, making choices based on core values, throat-moistening liquid foods, the thyroid gland, hearing/listening, and speech.

1. Do you know what you stand for?
2. Are you able to stay true to yourself even when your values are questioned?
3. Do you feel free to be you?
4. Do you appreciate that which makes you unique as a person?
5. Do you try your best to live in accordance with what you feel is important?
6. Do you speak your truth in a clear and conscientious way?
7. Are you comfortable expressing yourself verbally?
8. Do you find it easy to converse with others?
9. Are you able to speak as well as you can listen?
10. Do you speak up if there are issues about which you feel strongly?
11. Do you actively listen when someone else is speaking?
12. Can you effectively make a decision when you have too many choices?
13. Are you able to choose what is important to you?
14. Do you usually walk away knowing you made the best choice you could?
15. Are you comfortable making decisions?
16. Do you chew your food well?
17. Do you eat an adequate amount of food (not too little, not too much)?
18. Do you have a normal, healthy appetite?
19. When you eat, do you only eat and not multi-task?

20. Do you eat liquid foods regularly (e.g., soups, sauces, smoothies)?

21. Do you have a healthy sense of taste and smell?

22. Is your thyroid gland healthy, to the best of your knowledge?

23. Does your throat stay moist?

24. Do you have healthy teeth (e.g. no tooth loss)?

25. Is your jaw loose and relaxed?

Indigo/INSIGHT

This section of the quiz assesses your body, food, and life issues as they relate to the color **indigo (INSIGHT)** and its connection to **wisdom** in your life. These questions relate to the intellect/cognition, intuition, imagination, sleep, dreams, and mood.

1. Do you consider yourself to be smart or able to understand concepts easily?

2. Are you good at solving problems?

3. Do you find yourself thinking deeply about ideas or problems?

4. Do you like learning new things?

5. Are you a quick learner?

6. Are you intuitive?

7. Do you get impressions about things yet to happen?

8. Do you have a good sense of discernment?

9. Do you listen to your inner knowing?

10. Do your let your perceptions of a situation guide you through life events?

11. Do you sleep well through the night?

12. Do you regularly sleep seven to eight hours per night?

13. Do you have a consistent healthy sleep pattern?

14. Do you fall asleep easily without the use of sleep aids?

15. Do you wake in the morning feeling refreshed?

16. Do you avoid drinking too many caffeinated drinks?

17. Do you avoid eating too much chocolate?

18. Do you have a healthy relationship with food rather than feeling addicted?

19. Do you avoid drinking excessive amounts of alcoholic drinks?

20. Are you able to focus without relying on external substances (e.g., caffeine, alcohol)?

21. Are you able to clear your mind before bedtime?

22. Are you attentive to tasks on hand and mindful?

23. Is your memory good?

24. Are your moods stable?

25. Do you meditate or engage in a mindful practice of some sort?

White/SPIRIT

This section of the quiz assesses your body, food, and life issues as they relate to the color **white (SPIRIT)** and its connection to your **spiritual life**. It examines your sense of purpose and meaning, your faith, cleansing, purification, life force, and light.

1. Is your life full of meaning?

2. Do you feel connected to life in a spiritual way?

3. Are you concerned with greater global causes (e.g., ending hunger, world peace)?

4. Do you feel called to do certain things in your life?

5. Do you find yourself inspired to change the world in ways that you can?

6. Do you consider yourself a "spiritual" person?

7. Do you have faith that everything works out as it needs to be?

8. Do your spiritual views direct your life decisions at a high level?

9. Do you feel that you can withstand challenges because of your faith?

10. Do you believe in something greater than yourself?

11. Do you have regular exposure to sunlight?

12. Do you feel that you radiate an inner glow?

13. Do you sleep during the nighttime hours and stay awake during the daylight hours?

14. Do you have access to bright white lights in your living space?

15. Does life feel "light and wonderful" rather than "heavy and dark"?

16. Do you regularly cleanse your body through foods or fasting?

17. Do you take time to be quiet in prayer or meditation?

18. Do you eat fresh food rather than fried food?

19. Do you avoid plastic containers (e.g., for food, water, etc.)?

20. Do you avoid using toxic personal-care products (e.g., lotion, make-up, deodorant)?

21. Do you do what you can to minimize exposure to excessive electro-magnetic fields (EMFs)?

22. Is your nervous system healthy (e.g., no pain, numbness, etc.)?

23. Are you resilient; do you recover quickly from illness?

24. Do people say that you look younger than your age?

25. Do you think that your life force, or constitution, is stronger than most others'?

YOUR SPECTRUM QUIZ SCORE

Now that you have completed the Spectrum Quiz, you can calculate your Spectrum Quiz score in three simple steps:

1. Tally the number of "no" responses for each color:
   - Red/ROOT:
   - Orange/FLOW:
   - Yellow/FIRE:
   - Green/LOVE:
   - Aquamarine/TRUTH:
   - Indigo/INSIGHT:
   - White/SPIRIT:

2. Assess your number of "no" responses for each color.

- If you answered "no" to **fewer than ten statements** within any color, this color is likely to be balanced.

- If you answered "no" to **eleven to fifteen statements** within any color, you have a moderate imbalance of that color.

- If you answered "no" to **more than fifteen statements** within any color, you have a severe imbalance of that color.

- If your scores indicate that **all your colors are balanced** according to the numeric scale above, focus on the color(s) that had the highest number of "no" responses and make that your path forward.

3. You can read through the book in its entirety so you have a good idea of the overall approach, and then go back a second time to focus on the color that scored highest for you, or you can jump to the chapter of the system that reflects your highest (most imbalanced) score.

Your scores help you identify colors that include your core strengths, as well as colors that are out of balance. You'll learn more about each color within the Rainbow Diet in the next several chapters.

CHAPTER 3

EATING FOR YOUR INNER RAINBOW

Food is our common ground, a universal experience.

James Beard

Today, the average human body confronts an array of modern-day assaults: a nutrient-poor, calorie-excessive diet, little to no activity, exposure to environmental toxins, cigarette smoking, alcohol consumption, negative thinking, and perhaps significant emotional turmoil. No wonder we emerge from the daily battle feeling utterly fatigued, lifeless, and on the verge of breakdown. Our bodies may respond to these injuries by putting on extra weight to protect it. In the small sliver of time available before significant health issues arise, we often turn to rapid, quick-fix solutions to delay the onset of some of the symptoms.

In the midst of this whirlwind of stress on the body, we know that, deep within, we need to take the right actions to be healthy. Although we may know that we have to eat more vegetables and get more exercise, we may be so preoccupied and focused on getting through another day that we ignore those inner pleas.

We want to be vibrant, healthy, inspired, and full of bountiful energy to give to the thoughts, actions, and emotions that allow us to live our best lives. My experience and observations suggest that there are many paths to finding this freedom. One of them is through the vehicle of nourishment.

As human beings, we need external substances like food and water to keep us functioning optimally. In times of stress, we may need the help of specific nutrients to assist the cells with the necessary raw materials they require to harness sufficient energy and remove the accumulation of waste products. These substances enable the physical body to cope best with everyday events. When the physical body can flow and feel in control of its surroundings, it can free up more reserves to focus on its spiritual needs, including its life purpose and its connection with all of life.

We Are "Onioned" Beings

If you are reading this book, chances are you understand that a human being consists of several compressed layers, similar to those of an onion. Healing can occur by peeling away the layers. When we reach one layer—say, the emotional layer—and make a change, no matter how small or big, it ripples into every other aspect of our being, like a droplet of water losing itself in a pond. For seconds afterward, the pond is filled with the rhythmic beauty of concentric circles. Moreover, the composition of the pond has been changed forever because of that single, innocent droplet.

Food and nutrition are avenues that some people choose as paths to their healing. If you are especially drawn to diets and nutrition, it may simply be that food is what you need to get to where you need to be. No matter your choice of path, your journey will be symbolic for you in diverse ways. An underlying principle to remember throughout this book is that your relationship to food and eating is symbolic of how you approach everything else in your life. Do you eat convenience foods because you are always on the run? Well, then perhaps you need to reassess where your attention needs to be, or reconsider what you need to make time for. Or are you eating alone, secretly, especially if you are feeling emotional? If so, what needs to come out in the open? What needs expressing? With whom do you need to surround yourself?

Certainly, your relationship to food can open you up to insight about what your life is like. It has been said: "As within, so without"—in other words, our internal environment mirrors our external surroundings. Thus your restoration to wellness lies in your awareness of what envelops you, how you engage with the world, and how you interact with food and eating.

The impact that food choices can have on our health can be incredibly significant, especially due to the sheer quantity of food we eat throughout our lifetimes—estimated at 60,000 to 100,000 pounds! And we actually need all that just to exist on this planet. In fact, we are given many opportunities to make food selections that benefit the layers of our complex selves. A simple calculation of three meals a day, 365 days a year, for an average lifespan of seventy-six years means that we have almost 84,000 opportunities to have meaningful, healing interactions with food! There is unleashed potential in every single one of those interfaces. Each exchange carries the ability to bring us to a higher state of health, to keep us where we currently are, or to add to the pending avalanche of symptoms that culminate in disease.

In the grand theater of life, food takes center stage, as it serves our most primal need for survival, the bond we have with the Earth, and our intimate connections with each other. We fasten ourselves to the web of all living beings on the planet through the process of eating and being participants in the food chain. As a result, our incessant interaction with food takes on immense power and can define who we are. It is no wonder that people have strong opinions about how to eat.

Despite being constantly surrounded by food in all forms—from twenty-four-hour grocery stores to deluxe drive-thrus to vending machines—we ironically ignore its existence and our need for it. In the whirlwind of busy days, how many of us have thought to ourselves, or expressed to others, that having to eat "gets in the way" of doing more important things? Other people admit that they simply "forget" to eat. How can we neglect something so crucial to our survival? What message does this send forth? When we finally do make time to eat, we find ourselves unable to stop due to an unconscious longing for greater satisfaction and union in the midst of our hyperactive society and frequent fleeting social interactions with others. Yet with each hurried, unfulfilling bite, we step farther away from merging with everything with which food connects us—ourselves, our community, and nature.

Rather than experiencing a deeper level of understanding about foods and our bodies' need for growth and maintenance, we fixate on the path of least resistance, or short-term quick-fixes. Is it any wonder that the "diet" approach to eating is a rollercoaster of disappointment? Instead, we should be envisioning foods as dancing molecules of energy that have the power and potential to uncover our highest selves. We should make food choices that support life-giving thoughts, feelings, beliefs, and actions. Our lives can be revolutionized completely when we alter our view of food! And the beauty of this miracle is that it can start as soon as your next bite.

Fortunately, the eating revolution has begun. For example, the "slow food" movement, which encourages the longer, savory experience of eating a gradually cooked meal at a restaurant, has emerged as the antithesis to fast food. Local, organically grown foods and free-range, animal-sourced foods are becoming more prevalent. We are gradually returning to a very simple, yet profound, interaction with food.

Food Beyond the Calorie

Recently, we have come increasingly to recognize the power food has to affect us on many levels—physical, emotional, mental, and spiritual. Yet this power was recognized thousands of years ago by ancient traditions like Ayurvedic medicine and TCM. In both these traditions, balancing the energetic properties of different foods in the diet is strongly emphasized.

For example, in TCM, foods are selected according to their warming, cooling, drying, or moistening effects on the body. To the novice, it is relatively easy to select foods intuitively that embody certain properties, as the principles of the food parallel the concepts found in nature. In general, "warming" foods are those that "rev" the metabolism and create heat in the body, like spicy curried chicken. People with a "warm nature" or those who are prone to overheating should moderate their consumption of these foods. On the other hand, "cooling" foods are more neutral in taste and tend not to be cooked, like sliced cucumber or tofu. In contrast to "warming" foods, they dampen the metabolism, slowing it down.

Unfortunately, industrialized societies do not promote the use of foods to prevent disease as much as these traditions do. However, this trend is changing with the emergence of "functional medicine," or "integrative medicine," which acknowledges the inner communication between body systems and focuses on the individual as a whole.

Unlocking the Secret Messages of Food

Emerging science is shedding light on another angle of existing nutritional knowledge. In addition to providing energy, or calories, that allow the body to function, constituents within food act as messengers that communicate with your body's DNA and influence the types of protein and other compounds your cells manufacture. Taking this a step deeper, down to the atomic level, we now know that the charged particles of food interact electrically with the fluid matrix within the body to a significant degree. This tells us that food carries information that can either signal our bodies to create protein to support a vital, creative, optimal structure, or cause them to form dysfunctional states like inflammation and pain.

Nutritionists are taught in school that protein and carbohydrate both create the same energy currency within the body. For every gram of protein or carbohydrate eaten, four kilocalories of energy are made available for use. However, we now know that these basic nutrients, despite having similar caloric values, have different "informational signals." People can consume the same amount of calories of these foods, but experience different metabolic effects within their cells. Protein from vegetables—like soybeans—and protein from animals—like milk-derived casein—create different responses in the body because they contain different amino acids and other components like phytonutrients. For example, there may be certain proteins that help to reduce blood pressure more than others. Other proteins may have specific effects on neurotransmitters in the brain. The new realization is that the quality of food, and the dietary signature it carries for the cells, is perhaps most essential of all.

Unfortunately, it appears that the average diet has a deficit of good food signals. We are eating what I like to call the "brown, yellow, and white foods diet," which provides a limited supply of abundant, healthy compounds from plants ("phytochemicals") that equip our cells to work optimally. We are left with lackluster eating devoid of the rich, flavorful phytochemicals that send high-quality information to our cells, allowing us to flourish. Each compound of color, whether it's the purple anthocyanidins found in grapes or the red lycopene in tomatoes, has a specific function in the body. If we omit a color from the rainbow spectrum, we deny ourselves the full potential of what it can bring to our bodies and systems of health. As you will uncover in the chapters to come, "rainbow eating" is one of the keys to enhancing whole-self health.

Food Beyond the Body

In addition to the quality of our food, we also need to consider how a food is eaten. Think of all the health benefits of the Mediterranean diet. Do you think this region of Europe experiences fewer cardiovascular complications because they eat whole foods rich in precious plant compounds that are heart-protective and anti-aging? Most likely, but perhaps not entirely. One point that is often overlooked is the manner in which Mediterraneans eat. Meals for these people are often events potentially lasting for hours and carried out in the company of friends and family. Mealtimes in these countries are important social events, and working hours are adjusted to accommodate longer lunches. This flexibility enables individuals to go home to eat and relax before returning to work, all while grounding themselves in their ROOT and giving their bodies time to absorb essential nutrients. Imagine how little stress you would feel if you had one or two hours to eat lunch instead of thirty minutes. Think how that could impact your spectrum of responses to food!

Eating surely begins before and lasts after the first bite is taken. It starts in the grocery store when we are engaged in food selection, or as far back as in the field when we plant seeds in the soil. In the grocery store, what colors call out to you? What shapes, forms, tactile sensations, words on packages invite you to buy them? How mindful are you when you grocery shop? Are you distracted by cell-phone calls or mental preoccupation with the day's events? If you grow your own food, are you conscious of the quality of soil you use, your mindset when you water the plants, or where you plant seeds?

The process of eating continues to the stage of meal preparation, where you gift your olfactory sense with rich aromas and heightened flavors, eventually signaling your gastric juices to begin flowing and specific gut peptides for satiety to be released. If you make a meal with others, in a community setting, the quality of the experience expands many times, as it magnifies your interconnection with others. After the meal, the eating experience continues on a physiological level through the processes of digestion, absorption, and assimilation. If you eat quickly without mindfulness, you may not be efficient at integrating these food messages into your body and soul. Without a sense of pleasure and being present in the moment of eating, you may want to eat more to satisfy your need to connect with the experience. Therefore, eating while doing other things—driving a car, watching TV, or reading a book—may take away healing energy from the eating experience, rather than providing it.

Quantum "Phoods"

Modern physics gives a whole new twist to how we view living matter. Essentially, all living organisms are compositions of cosmic, dynamic, responsive particles vibrating at a specific frequency. It has been said that the building block of life, the atom, is made of more than 90 percent empty space, implying that only about 10 percent of what is recognized as an organism is actual physical matter. The majority of any life form is really vibrating energy. These particles of dancing matter form a web of connection, sending signals and creating patterns, vortices, and cascading effects. When we think of ourselves as molecules in motion, it is highly plausible that the frequency generated by these interacting particles is modified by our thoughts, our words, the air we breathe, and even the food we eat. Many published research studies on meditation, prayer, visualization, and diet support the idea that our minds, words, and environment can influence our emotional, mental, and physical make-up.

The fact that foods have different subtle effects is not entirely new. Ayurveda classifies foods promoting purity and vitality as *sattvic*. These foods are not "expensive" for the body to process and they do not leave behind harmful toxins. They are described as "savory, smooth, firm, and pleasant to the stomach," in contrast to foods that are *rajasic*, or "excessively pungent, sour, salty, hot, harsh, astringent, and burnt" and can lead to sickness. Examples of sattvic foods include those that are mild, cooling, and refreshing—fruits, vegetables, raw milk, clarified butter (known as *ghee*), and honey. Meats are perceived as rajasic, as the flesh is thought to harbor the fear and anger of the animal that was killed, transferring it to the eater.

In modern society, some foods are considered toxic. These are foods that have been damaged through their processing—by overcooking, burning, mechanical overprocessing, and oxidation. Interestingly, recent scientific studies have shown that foods that have been browned through cooking can age and inflame our cells. Acrylamide and rancid fat are examples of toxic compounds that form in products like potato chips when the potato slices are heated in oil. Likewise, leftover meals may seem convenient, but they are often devoid of any life-giving energy.

Food is dynamic, living, and responsive to external attitudes, thoughts, words, and actions. We add to the quality of foods through our thoughts, intentionally bumping up or eroding the healing, transformative potential that is part of the food. If you are eating a lush, green leafy salad with a head full of toxic thoughts, I just don't believe that you are reaping the full benefits of the meal. Similarly, eating a fast-food hamburger with a mindful attitude isn't a complete picture either. I have observed that, by putting your intention into food, you interact much more deeply with it during eating. If you hold positive, good thoughts while eating, your physiology and psychology may be altered so that the food particles are digested and absorbed in ways that are beneficial.

Eating with Consciousness

My motto is this: To reap the benefits of food, be present in its presence. In fact, this point may be even more essential than the actual food itself. Although the substance the food provides is important, the attention we bring into the process of eating it may be equally important.

Our conscious relationship to food begins the moment we choose it, whether at the grocery store, the farmer's market, or in a restaurant. This process involves appreciating and giving gratitude for every step involved in the production of the food, thereby honoring its sacredness. The act of eating food is unifying because it connects us to all of life. The gratitude we express for a plant or animal giving up its energy for the sake of our own is woven into our evolution as conscious beings. When we chew our food, it is imperative that we be present in that experience, knowing that we are participating in the process of transforming energy. Each bite captures the entire lineage of the food, from a gross level of physiological breakdown, to raw energy for use by the cells, to the finer essence of what was brought to the food by the people involved in growing, manufacturing, harvesting, choosing, and preparing it. Every morsel contains something more than calories that we can tap into if we are fully present in the moment of our interaction and exchange with food.

CHAPTER 4

SUPPLEMENTS

Millions of Americans today are taking dietary supplements, practicing yoga and integrating other natural therapies into their lives. These are all preventive measures that will keep them out of the doctor's office and drive down the costs of treating serious problems like heart disease and diabetes.

Andrew Weil, MD

Food and supplements can work well together. One point I would like to emphasize, however, is that supplements are not a quick fix for chronic, deep-rooted issues. They are also not a replacement for a healthy diet. They are best used in collaboration with a number of therapeutic modalities. Symptoms and disease can be tackled with a variety of tactics. Some are physical—like food, supplements, and activity. Others are emotional—like therapy, journaling, and creative expression. By drawing on multiple resources, we are better positioned to be more effective in tackling the issues at hand and preparing ourselves for a shift in the direction of healing.

A variety of supplement products—capsules, creams, granules, jellies, liquids, patches, powders, wafers, and the like—are widely available at health food stores, supermarkets, and pharmacies. Not all of them are equal when it comes to quality, however. The contents of some supplements may be questionable. There may be discrepancies in dose, either too much or too little, that go unnoticed. There is also the risk that the supplement is contaminated with a substance that was not intended to be in the final product. Ensure that you purchase your natural products from a reputable source, preferably a healthcare professional.

Once you purchase your supplements, remember that they are only as effective as the degree to which their potency is preserved. Protect their potency by storing them in the manner that is optimal. Some of them will be susceptible to breaking down in the presence of heat, light, and/or air. For example, probiotics (healthy bacteria for the gut) are usually refrigerated to keep the bacteria alive. B vitamins degrade rapidly in the presence of heat, light, and exposure to oxygen, so they need to be kept in a cool, dark place. Guidance on how to keep the supplement is typically provided on its label. If not, ask your healthcare professional or read literature on that supplement. On the product itself, you will also find an expiration date. Do not use supplements that are older than their expiration date, as you may not receive their full benefit. In some cases, they could break down into other compounds that are not necessarily good for the body. For instance, fish oil that is kept too long or is left to degrade may develop a "fishy" odor, indicating that it has become rancid.

Macronutrients

The word "macronutrients" designates nutrients we need to eat in relatively large (macro) quantities, usually in gram amounts. These include the nutrient trio of carbohydrate, fat, and protein. Of course, since we need these nutrients in bulk, we often eat enough in our diet, although perhaps not always in the ideal proportion. There may be times you need special forms of these macronutrients, like a powdered fiber supplement (nondigestible carbohydrate) to support the movement of the gut, or a fish oil capsule to help you get the right proportion of essential fat. These three macronutrients form the core of the physical body by giving it an underlying structural foundation and basic functioning capacity.

Protein

The foundation of the body relies on the solid, durable structure of protein. Proteins are highly organized macronutrients that can be disassembled into their amino-acid building blocks. They are used for supporting muscle and building antibodies to keep the body protected from outside invaders, and hormones and enzymes. Essentially, your body would be jelly without the framework of protein to hold it all together. Protein allows you to have a structure to ground to the Earth, giving your body the ability to be stable, yet in motion. There are about twenty amino acids that are essential and must be eaten in the diet. Your body can also make a variety of (non-essential) amino acids. Various types of supplement protein powders are available; soy, whey, rice, pea, and hemp are some of the popular ones.

Fat

Fat is an underestimated, undervalued macronutrient. Unfortunately, the food industry has encouraged some degree of "fat phobia" with the multitude of "fat-free" products introduced in the 1990s. As a result, people are skeptical about eating this essential nutrient. It is unique from other macronutrients in that it is the most concentrated source of energy (one gram of fat yields nine calories versus the four calories from carbohydrate and protein), which is likely the root of its bad reputation. Fat is pervasive in the body. Every cell in the body needs a membrane made of fat, and most of brain tissue is fat.

Within the fat nutrient group, there are two main types: saturated fat (generally animal-based fat, but also tropical oils like coconut and palm oil) and unsaturated fat (typically plant-based fat). The body cannot make certain unsaturated fats, like omega-6 and omega-3, so they have been coined "essential fats," meaning that we must eat them. If we don't eat enough of these fats relative to other dietary fats, eyes, skin, hair, and nails suffer. Vision can worsen as well, while the skin can become rough, hair can fall out, and nails can fray. Due to the high quantity of these fats in the brain, they are also important for behavior. You can't concentrate or feel good without them. Supplemental forms of fat include fish oil (high in omega-3 fats called eicosapentaenoic acid, or "EPA," and docosahexaenoic acid, "DHA"), flaxseed oil, borage oil, and evening primrose oil.

Carbohydrate

The majority of what most people eat (40–60 percent of calories) is carbohydrate, a macronutrient used primarily for energy (glucose). Carbohydrates are the rescuer nutrients—like mini life-preservers, they come into the body and give it a quick burst of energy. The problem is that you can't live your life eating quick-fix carbohydrates every time you feel your energy waning. Rather, you must learn to shift your eating to long-term, sustained change. Fortunately, there is a way to do that with the help of carbohydrates. Carbohydrates are divided into two categories: simple and complex. Simple carbohydrates encompass simple sugars like sucrose (white table sugar), fructose (fruit sugar), and lactose (milk sugar). These can give you a quick burst of energy, followed by a crash. Complex carbohydrates are longer chains of sugars. Some of them cannot be digested and absorbed (fibers), while others can (starches). Complex carbohydrates generally provide you with longer-lasting, sustainable energy, especially when paired with soluble fiber, like psyllium-seed husk.

Micronutrients

Micronutrients are on the opposite end of the spectrum. They are required in relatively smaller amounts, compared with macronutrients. Instead of grams, we may only need 1/1000th of a gram (known as a microgram, or mcg) to fulfill our bodily needs. Vitamins and minerals fall into this category of nutrient. They can serve as the helpers for the macronutrients and as catalysts for a number of processes. For example, protein provides amino acids like tryptophan, which can be transformed into the neurotransmitter serotonin if vitamin B6 is present in adequate quantities. Similarly, zinc is needed to convert small-chain essential fat into long-chain fat needed for the brain and eyes. Although they are typically needed in smaller amounts, their importance to the body is not diminished.

Vitamin and mineral deficiencies tend to be more common in times of stress, war, or impoverishment. Ironically, however, in our industrialized world, people are still starving for adequate amounts of quality nutrients—particularly micronutrients. The U.S. Food and Drug Administration (FDA) has established recommendations for the intake of micronutrients to prevent deficiency, tailored for gender and age. You can find these recommendations on their website at *ods.od.nih.gov.* Bear in mind, however, that these recommendations do not take into account those who have special needs—for example, those with genetic variability, those on limited diets or on prescription medications, or those who smoke or drink alcohol.

Supplements containing vitamins and minerals are easy to locate in a number of stores, and they can come in the form of a single, active at a high dose, or in combination. It is important to recognize that high doses of a single vitamin or mineral may offset levels of another vitamin or mineral and may potentially create an imbalance or relative deficiency. Along similar lines, some micronutrients work better as a team. The family of B vitamins acts together in the process of extracting energy from macronutrients like carbohydrates.

Vitamins and Minerals

Vitamins are required in small amounts to assist overall body processes, like helping the body to digest and metabolize macronutrients. The family of vitamins is divided into two classes: fat-soluble and water-soluble. For the most part, in order for the body to take in fat-soluble vitamins optimally, they need to be accompanied by a source of fat. These vitamins are usually retained in the body for a longer period of time in the fat tissue. Fat-soluble vitamins include A, D, E, and K.

On the other hand, water-soluble vitamins are absorbed readily, without fat. However, they also leave the body quickly through conduits of water like sweat and urine. These vitamins include the B vitamins (thiamin, riboflavin, niacin, pantothenic acid, pyridoxine, folic acid, cyanocobalamin) and vitamin C.

Minerals are similar to vitamins in that only small amounts are needed in the body for maintenance of body pH—the amount of acidity and alkalinity in body compartments, which is very tightly controlled. They also regulate the formation of bone and blood, nervous-system function, muscular contraction and release, and normal enzyme function.

There is a natural division among minerals. Some of them are required in larger amounts (several hundred milligrams, or even slightly more than a gram), like calcium, magnesium, potassium, and phosphorus. Others are needed in tiny trace amounts, like chromium, copper, iodine, manganese, selenium, and zinc. Vitamins and minerals can both be obtained from foods; however, minerals usually come from within the Earth's crust. Plants incorporate these minerals from the soil, and are ultimately eaten by humans or by animals.

Herbs

Herbs have been used since ancient times to cure a host of diseases. Available scientific research suggests that the inner workings of plants may be more complex than that of human beings. There is the perception that herbs have healing properties and, since they are "natural," they can be used indiscriminately. However, this is not the case. As mentioned, they are very potent substances. They can deliver health benefits when employed wisely, but can be counter-productive when used unwisely. You must be cautious when using herbs, just as you exercise caution when taking a pharmaceutical.

In supplement form, there are many ways to use herbs internally:

- **Decoctions**: The bark, berry, root, or seed of a plant is made into a tea preparation.

- **Extracts**: The herb is pressed mechanically and soaked in water or alcohol. Then the liquid it was soaked in is allowed to evaporate.

- **Powders**: The herb is ground into a powder and then delivered in a capsule or tablet.

- **Tinctures**: The herb is preserved in liquid, usually alcohol, but sometimes in a non-alcohol form like glycerin.

CHAPTER 5

THE RED ROOT

I think that what we're seeking is an experience of being alive, so that our life experiences on the purely physical plane will have resonances within our own innermost being and reality, so that we can actually feel the rapture of being alive.

Joseph Campbell

KEY WORDS FOR THE ROOT: ancestors, being present, blood, body, Earth, family/tribe, grounded, instinct, nature, origins, physical matter, protection, red, security, survival

Why does it sometimes take so long to make a shift in your body, behaviors, actions, and thoughts? You can thank your ROOT for the slow steadiness of your change! The ROOT is the part of you that is grounded in the workings of the physical world and represents stability, certainty, and physical strength. It is the foundation of your identity. Being grounded simply means being present in your body in every moment, from head to toe. When you feel this connection to your physical body, your awareness of the surrounding environment is enhanced, making for fewer accidents and inefficiencies. As a result, your life feels full and under control.

The ROOT system provides much of the framework for the other colors of your inner spectrum. It can be compared to laying the physical foundation for the "house" of who you are. Without a firm foundation and established layers of trust, security, and safety, you can easily crumble under pressure.

The ROOT and Your Body

The ROOT system is the instinctual, primal template for who you are as a physical human being. It represents your physical structure, and includes your joints, bones, muscles, legs, and feet. It also equips you with an internal and external defense system. The immune system is your internal "defense" strategy, while your skin is your external "defense" strategy—a physical barrier that separates you from environmental influences, your self from your non-self. This defense system provides you with healthy boundaries.

Adding to boundaries and defending the self are the adrenal glands. They are like the internal armory that provides you with the ability to "fight" or "flee" if you are in a situation that threatens your life. The adrenals give you that instinctual, primal urge to live no matter the cost and to make that decision instantaneously. That instinct to survive is hardwired into you on the DNA level. The ROOT system also represents the red and white blood cells, products of the bone marrow, and your identity that is carried within every cell in the form of your double-stranded DNA. Your DNA and immune system allow you to know who you are and are not.

The ROOT and Eating

Since the ROOT focuses primarily on the part of you that needs basic elements for survival, it is closely tied to your relationship with food and eating. Therefore, it is not surprising that your food issues are contained within the earthy terrain of this system of health. Here are some simple questions you can ask yourself to determine if you are maintaining a balanced ROOT.

Do you feel secure?
Without air, food, and water, you are without life. Money provides the abundance to access food. The way you "earn a living" and your feelings about money are directly related to your ROOT system. If you have an imbalance in this area, you may feel an absence of abundance. Someone

who is stingy with the money spent on meals or someone who fixates on and becomes preoccupied with the money spent on food may have a ROOT system that requires healing.

It works the other way, too. An imbalance in the ROOT can result if you are obsessive to the point of maximizing buffets and "getting your money's worth" from an open selection of foods. For example, in social settings, Jim deliberately eats what remains on everyone else's plate at the end of a shared meal to ensure that all the food is gone and not wasted. Similarly, Jillian comes from a large family where food was scarce, and admits that she does not feel safe unless her pantry is completely stocked full. Creating a healthy ROOT system involves releasing ingrained fear messages about providing and eating food and the security it brings to your physical existence. Instead, redirect your focus toward cultivating a sense of safety inside yourself.

Do you eat only when you are hungry?

In my opinion, one of the biggest problems with eating behavior in modern society is that we no longer rely on the body's instinct. We don't seem to trust our impulses about what we need to eat. Instead, we look to books on "how to eat" to tell us what we need. We ask the wait staff at a restaurant what's the best thing on the menu. Sometimes, we even give up our right to choose our foods by having others cook or order for us on a routine basis.

Neglecting your body's needs by removing choice or denying yourself foods indicates that your ROOT system needs work. Self-inflicted starvation and anorexia, for example, are classic examples of the physical, grounded nature of a ROOT system in need of deep healing. When you refuse food, your body form becomes almost non-existent and withers to a willowy, thin shell. Food becomes an enemy rather than a nourishing, supportive substance. Individuals who refuse to eat have difficulty accepting that they have the "right to exist"—a major cornerstone of the ROOT.

Another ROOT issue arises when you are out of touch with your body and unable to distinguish between emotional and physical hunger. Physical hunger comes from the ROOT of survival and originates deep within you—in contrast to emotional hunger, which springs from the FLOW part of you, as you will read in the next chapter. Physical hunger is a very distinct signal that builds gradually and is open to a variety of food choices. Frequently, your body's signals are not heard clearly enough because you do not pay attention and mistake your emotional food needs for physical hunger.

SAFE-PLACE IMAGERY AND PHYSICAL HUNGER

Your ROOT encompasses what it means to have healthy physical hunger and to be able to honor that sensation when you feel the urge. When you ignore or confuse your body's hunger signals, you refuse to place trust in your body. By dialoguing with your body about the foods it needs, you can fulfill your physical needs and satisfy your ROOT system. The dialogue may be as simple as walking into your kitchen, feeling your toes on the floor to ground yourself, and asking your body what you need to eat. Sometimes, I recommend that people cultivate a "safe place" within. This can be some body part that you go to in order to connect fully to what is happening within you—like an internal ally. See what kinds of activities are happening in your safe place. Are there messages, symbols, or signs? Perhaps, a special color or feeling when you know something is right? When you practice this technique, you develop a better trusting relationship with your body in the moment. Eventually, you will react appropriately to signals that your body is hungry, rather than suppressing or ignoring them.

Do you try to protect yourself with food?

Currently, more than 60 percent of the population in industrialized countries has been categorized as overweight or obese. No apparent solution exists for this growing crisis. Of course, there are many contributors to excess body weight, including lifestyle behaviors like eating poorly and remaining sedentary. However, if we look deeper to unearth the real causes, we may find that excess weight for some individuals may be linked to their inability to feel safe. The added weight provides padding and protection from attention. Julie admits that she started to gain weight as a teenager after people commented on the changes in her body and how attractive she was becoming. Her feelings of being scared and intimidated by the changes in her body turned into overeating. During our nutrition consultation, Julie reflected on the power that these comments, made to her some forty years ago, continue to have over her.

Other clients have revealed to me that they have been physically or sexually abused in their lives. As a result, they feel safer when they cover their bodies with excess weight so no one can see their true form. Just like not eating enough, eating too much involves the ROOT system. Too much eating can unground you just as much as not eating at all. You numb yourself when you take in too much food, causing yourself to let go of feeling. When you do not eat at all, you do not have the strength to feel, process thoughts and emotions, and be active. In both cases, you eject yourself from your body through the mechanism of food.

Instead of hiding yourself in the shadow of too much food, you can use food to bring out the best in you—the vital, pure essence of who you are, basking in love. When you eat according to your body's needs, your mind remains sharp and your heart strong. You can focus on the moment and give attention to any thoughts, words, or actions that float in your sky of consciousness, allowing you to feel alive and connected!

Do you engage in healthy social eating?

Social eating is a charged event. Most often, especially around the holidays, people tell me that they are conflicted by social eating events. Sometimes, they teeter on the stressful decision of whether to attend a gathering because of the foods that may be served. They find it fearful to challenge the tribe aspects of eating by refusing certain foods. Alexandra told me how, at a party, a brownie was thrust into her mouth by a family member before she could say "no." Later that day, she ended up with a throbbing migraine, as chocolate is one of her trigger foods. She was bedridden for hours. Even though she knew this would be the outcome, she was unable to find the internal strength to trust her own instinct and body, and go against her eating tribe.

When it comes to the ROOT system, there are different strategies you can use for dealing with challenging social aspects—for example, eating before the event, calling ahead of time to find out what will be served, or even participating in the tribal preparation of a meal by bringing a healthy dish!

Eating Activities for the ROOT

1. What belief patterns about food and eating did you inherit from your family? Are these belief patterns still valid for you? If not, list the new belief patterns. List the eating traditions and beliefs you wish to keep. Cultivate these with a fresh start.

2. Experience the process of how food is grown. Visit a farm and learn about farming practices. Buy a package of seeds; plant them in soil. Eat the food that you grow. How is your experience of eating made different by doing so?

3. Eat close to the earth, on the ground, barefoot one time per day. Write about whether or how this changes your eating experience.

4. Note when foods make you feel "grounded" and "ungrounded."

5. Practice checking in with your body on food choices. What language does your body use to tell you what and when to eat and when to stop eating?

6. Eat a meal using your hands that you wouldn't normally eat that way. Have fun!

7. Create a community of individuals who eat together based on a shared perspective of food and eating.

8. Draw your body on a piece of paper. Ask someone you trust to give you feedback on your drawing. Is it accurate? What observations do they note? Set an intention for a healthy body image and for greater acceptance of the gift of your flesh.

Foods for Your ROOT

There are certain foods that can help you re-establish and strengthen your connection with your body, making you feel heavy and slower-moving, grounding you to the often hectic world. These grounding foods give you the "earthly substance" you need to keep your feet on the Earth and to make your dreams real and practical. They are ideal for enabling you to be centered and protected when you walk the line between distraction and vulnerability.

Protein

Protein is a primary nutrient that gives you your physical structure. The building blocks of protein (amino acids) are contained throughout the physical structure of your body, in muscle, bone, and the immune system. If we zoom in closer to the cellular level, we see that protein is responsible for many of the minute happenings within the cell, such as catalyzing reactions, and maintaining cell shape and growth. They serve as the chief implementers of the information that is encoded in your genes.

Of the twenty or so amino acids that exist and are arranged in protein in various combinations, about eight are considered essential for your existence. Your physical body cannot manufacture these on its own—they simply must be eaten. A full complement of the essential amino acids is found in animal foods. Foundational, grounding high-protein foods include eggs and milk. Think of the nature of a hen's egg. If it were fertilized, it would have all the necessary nutritional constituents for nourishing the growth of a chick embryo. Animal-based foods are usually higher in complete protein than most other vegetable-based foods. However, that doesn't mean that they are necessarily better for you. They come with some downsides as well. They often contain growth hormone, antibiotics, and fat-loving environmental toxins. If you do eat animal protein, choose lean and clean (organic, pasture-raised, wild-caught) options to maximize the protein content.

Despite the fact that it is easier to get high-quality protein from animal-based foods, they can also be obtained from vegetable protein sources like legumes, nuts, and seeds. Usually, a combination of these vegetable foods is needed to get the same amino acid spectrum available in animal-based foods—for instance, the famous rice-and-beans combination. However, complementing vegetable protein is not always needed. Some proteins, like soy, are complete enough to stand alone—but be sure to choose high-quality, organic soy if you choose to eat it! The scientific debate continues over whether vegetable protein is preferable to animal protein for indications such as heart disease, hypertension, and cancer. Personally, I use vegetable protein like legumes, nuts, and seeds as a constant grounding baseline for most individuals, but not everyone can tolerate these foods. Some folks may prefer and feel drawn to animal protein for various reasons. It is best to be in tune with your body (your ROOT!) to read these needs specifically.

Protein-containing foods are a staple of every meal in many countries. However, eating primarily protein without a balance of the other macro-nutrients can wreak havoc in the body. An excess of animal protein and a deficiency of fruits and vegetables can lead to an imbalance of pH in the body systems, resulting in greater acid load. It is important to balance pH in the body, because numerous reactions in cells take place at specific pH ranges. For example, the enzymes that break down protein in the stomach function best at a low (acidic) pH, while the enzymes that break down starches in the small intestine work at a slightly alkaline pH. Greater acid milieu can throw the body out of balance and change the function of many organs. When there is high acid due to the intake of protein-rich, animal foods (composed of amino *acids*) without the buffering of fruits and vege-tables, the body reads that as a signal to borrow from its precious alkaline reserves to normalize the levels. Increased body acidity has the potential to steal alkalizing minerals (namely calcium) from tissues like the bones in order to bring the body back to a normal pH range. As a result, your bones may become brittle and susceptible to breaking. Measuring urine pH periodically is a good way to test how acidic you are so that you can adjust your eating accordingly.

USDA recommended servings of selected animal and vegetable pro-tein sources are given in Table 1. For more details, go to the USDA Nutri-ent Database at *nal.usda.gov*.

Minerals

While protein is important for your body, it is also important not to forget essential micronutrients, which are found in your diet in smaller amounts (1,000 or 1,000,000 times smaller than a gram!). Symbolically, minerals like calcium, iron, and zinc are all found deep in the layers of the Earth's crust, giving the Earth a strong physical structure. In much the same way, these minerals endow you with a bodily structure and framework so that many of your inner workings run smoothly. Interestingly, some studies have shown that organic food provides higher levels of minerals (as well as

TABLE 1. PROTEIN LEVELS OF SELECT ANIMAL AND VEGETABLE FOODS

Food	Serving	Weight in Grams	Protein Grams
Cheddar cheese	1 oz	28	7.1
Chicken, roasted	6 oz	170	42.5
Egg	1 large	50	6.3
Hamburger, extra lean	6 oz	170	48.6
Lentils, cooked	½ cup	99	9
Tofu	½ cup	126	10.1
Tuna, water-packed	6 oz	170	40.1
Yogurt, low-fat	8 oz	227	11.9

vitamins) compared with conventional food. Make sure to include these essential nutrients in your diet.

Calcium

A large majority—about 99 percent—of the calcium in your body is stored in your bone and teeth structures. Calcium helps to balance your overall body pH so that your cellular reactions can flow optimally. Excessive calcium, under certain conditions, can lead to the calcification of organs, like the kidneys.

Iron

This mineral is necessary for healthy red-blood-cell formation. Much of the bioavailable iron is present in animal foods like red meat, fish, and poultry. However, iron is also found in some vegetable foods, like lentils and beans. Vitamin C works well with iron and, in some cases, can help your body process more iron from foods. Try adding lemon juice to a spinach salad to harness the power of this combination.

Zinc

Zinc has a strong reputation as an essential element, as it is needed for thousands of reactions in the body involving protein. Like iron, zinc is primarily found in animal foods.

Root Vegetables

If there were just one food that would nourish the earthy ROOT part of you, root vegetables would be the logical candidate. The idea of the ROOT system going together with root vegetables is not far-fetched. Root vegetables are tough, solid, and durable. In nature's perfectly planned way, root vegetables support your own ROOT, which is attempting to do the same thing—keep you tough, durable, and able to weather survival issues.

Root vegetables are relatively rich sources of fiber and have necessary soil minerals that assist in the structure and function of organs ruled by the ROOT system. Tough, insoluble fibers provide you with bulk and solidness, cleansing your body of foreign material or toxins that get trapped in their network along the way. They enable you to have the sensation of being whole and full of substance, similar to the healthy feeling of being centered and grounded.

Aside from fiber, root vegetables supply some essential minerals (selenium, iron, magnesium, potassium) that are crucial for the process of cellular growth and the development of structural tissues. For example, magnesium is stored largely in muscle and bones, and it is necessary for, among other things, muscle relaxation, neuromuscular activity, and protein synthesis. Similarly, potassium is an electrolyte used for a variety of functions, like muscle contraction and maintenance of cell integrity.

Here are some root vegetables that can supply fiber and essential minerals to balance your ROOT:

Beets
Burdock
Carrots
Celery Root
Daikon
Garlic
Ginger root
Horseradish
Leek
Parsnips
Radish
Rutabaga

Shallots
Taro
Turnip
Wasabi
Yam
Yucca

Red-Colored Foods

While *red* meat is the clear choice for a protein-rich, ROOT-supporting food for those who eat meat, there are many other foods that offer other ROOT-supporting nutrients. Red plants like beets, tomatoes, cranberries, raspberries, strawberries, pomegranate, and apples provide relatively high levels of vitamin C and plant nutrients referred to as polyphenols. These two compounds serve the body in a general sense as antioxidants, or part of cellular and bodily defense. They work to clean up cellular debris and to quench reactive radicals that perpetuate cell damage. Lycopene is one of the plant compounds in red foods that make it red. It is one of the most potent, protective antioxidants, and has been shown to be beneficial in the prevention and treatment of cancer and cardiovascular disease.

Vitamin C is not only an effective antioxidant; it also boasts several other functions essential to being grounded. Vitamin C helps the collagen matrix form, thereby supporting structures like bone, teeth, and skin. Vitamin C is also important for the health of the immune system and adrenal glands.

Here are some examples of red-colored fruits that support a balanced ROOT system:

Apples (Fuji, Pink Lady, Red Delicious)
Blood orange
Cherries
Cranberries
Nectarines
Pink grapefruit
Pomegranate
Raspberries
Red currants

Red pears
Red plums
Strawberries
Watermelon

Likewise, these red-colored vegetables are effective as part of the cellular and bodily defense provided by the ROOT:

Beets
Radishes
Red bell peppers
Red cabbage
Red chard
Red jalapeno pepper
Red onion
Red potatoes
Tomato-based products (e.g., sun-dried tomato, tomato paste, tomato sauce, salsa)
Tomatoes (e.g., vine-ripened, cherry)

And, of course, the primary source of ROOT support from animal products, should you choose them, comes from good old "red meat," or beef.

Supplements for Your ROOT

While it is always best to get nutrients for your ROOT from a diet containing protein, minerals, insoluble fiber, and red-colored foods, you may need to supplement with nutrients at various times when you need more support. In this section, I talk about supplements for the ROOT, which include protein powders, insoluble fiber, vitamins and minerals, herbs, and phytonutrients.

Protein Powders

Most of the protein you consume is obtained through your diet—through meat, yogurt, milk, cheese, beans, and nuts. With increasing rates of food intolerance and allergy (both ROOT-based health issues, by the way), we may need to avoid certain dietary proteins; yet, at the same time, we have to make sure we have sufficient protein. Here's where the use of high-quality, protein-based supplement powders like rice, soy, pea, and whey can come in handy. When you need a pick-me-up for your ROOT, try drinking a shake made in the blender using protein powder that suits your body and red fruits like raspberries or strawberries.

Stomach bloating immediately or shortly after eating protein may suggest that you are not fully digesting your dietary protein. As you advance in age, your stomach tends to make less hydrochloric acid, a strong acid produced in the stomach to denature and digest protein. Without this acid, your ability to digest and take in protein is significantly impaired. The undigested food in your stomach can result in its fermentation, and the subsequent bloating that brings.

For those with low stomach-acid production (a condition referred to as hypochlorhydria) or an absence of stomach acid (called achlorhydria), hydrochloric acid (HCl) supplements are useful. In some cases, these can be beneficial for individuals with food allergies and autoimmune disease like rheumatoid arthritis. HCl supplements are usually found as betaine HCl—with betaine as a carrier for the HCl. You must be very careful in how you take an HCl supplement, however. For example, these should not be taken with an NSAID (e.g., aspirin, ibuprofen) or corticosteroid (e.g., prednisone), since the combination may cause severe gastric upset. Betaine HCl in tablet or capsule form should be taken mid-way through a large, protein-containing meal. There are various recommendations on dosage. You can start at the minimum dose (600 mg) and see whether you experience less bloating and stomach upset. If not, try gradually increasing the dosage until you experience symptom relief. Taking too much betaine HCl can lead to a sharp heartburn sensation. These supplements are contraindicated if you have an ulcer or reflux.

If you struggle with protein digestion, it is also important to take a look outside of your body. Take note of what may be particularly difficult to digest in terms of information relating to your family of origin, your job, or making ends meet. When you feel overwhelmed by your circumstances relating to survival, you may not be able to digest your protein sources efficiently. When you do not get enough protein because of indigestion, you may experience delayed wound healing, hair loss, immune impairment, skin roughness or inflammation, and muscle breakdown.

Insoluble Fiber

Insoluble fiber, or the type of chewy fiber that speeds the passage of foods through your digestive tract, is helpful in ensuring healthy bowel movements and, therefore, the release of toxins. Without enough fiber in your diet, you may be prone to constipation and hemorrhoids. Dietary supplement powders containing insoluble fibers—for example, cellulose, oat bran, or rice bran—are beneficial for this purpose. It is advisable to take supplemental fiber separate from other supplements (especially minerals) or medications, because the fiber can potentially bind the actives and prevent their absorption in the gut.

Vitamins and Minerals

A wide variety of vitamins and minerals are available to support your ROOT system. Minerals, in fact, play a key role in stabilizing the ROOT system and comprise an important overall category of nutrients for the ROOT. Here are just a few of the more important vitamins and minerals, along with information for their safe use.

Vitamin A

Vitamin A, or retinol, is a fat-soluble vitamin commonly found in animal foods like meat, eggs, and whole milk.

- **Functions:** When taken orally, vitamin A can improve the immune system, skin and mucosal surfaces, cell division and growth, bone development, eye health, and embryonic development. It may also play a role in inhibiting cancer development. It is used in topical applications for skin-health benefits (reducing wrinkles, UV protection, and wound healing).

- **Deficiency:** Lack of vitamin A can lead to decreased immune function, night blindness that can develop into vision loss if not treated, and increased risk of infection.

- **Overuse:** Short-term, high doses (15,000 mcg, or 50,000 units) can cause nausea, vomiting, headache, spinal pressure, and blurred vision. Taking greater than or equal to 30,000 mcg (100,000 units) for long periods of time (months, years) can result in liver toxicity, fatigue, irritability, drastic behavioral changes, nausea, vomiting, and itchy, red skin. Too much vitamin A can also have a negative effect on bones. Intakes of greater than or equal to 10,000 units daily have been shown to increase risk for osteoporosis and hip fractures in postmenopausal women.

- **Interactions:** Caution is needed when taking vitamin A together with drugs that can negatively impact liver function. Avoid concomitant use with retinoids and with anti-coagulant supplements and drugs.

- **Relationship to the ROOT:** Vitamin A supports essential ROOT functions by regulating immunity and promoting skin integrity.

Vitamin B9

Vitamin B9 is commonly known as folic acid. The word "folate" derives from *folium*, which means "leaf" in Latin. Folate is a water-soluble vitamin present in a wide variety of foods, including leafy green vegetables. It is also present in fruits, whole grains, legumes, and some meats. The supplemental form of folate, referred to as folic acid, is found in supplements and processed foods.

- **Functions:** Since this vitamin assists in the formation of red and white blood cells, it is important for preventing anemia and for maintaining healthy immune function. It is a core nutrient required for healthy cell division and growth. Because of its role in protein metabolism, folic acid, together with vitamins B6 and B12, converts the amino acid homocysteine into non-harmful amino acids in the body. Elevated homocysteine has been shown to be associated with increased incidence of atherosclerosis (blood vessel narrowing due to build-up of plaque). Folate/folic acid intake is important for pregnant women, particularly early in pregnancy, because it is needed for embryonic and fetal nerve-cell development.

- **Intake:** High doses of folic acid should not be taken for extended periods if a hormone-sensitive cancer or seizure disorder is present.

- **Deficiency:** Lack of folic acid may result in anemia, fatigue, gastro-intestinal upset, sore or red tongue, growth impairment, insomnia, memory problems, paranoia, weakness, and birth defects.

- **Overuse:** Folic acid has relatively low toxicity, but high doses can result in abdominal cramps, diarrhea, rash, altered sleep patterns, and neurological disturbances. Daily doses of 1000 mcg should not be exceeded to prevent folate from masking a deficiency of vitamin B12.

- **Interactions:** This supplement may interfere with the actions of methotrexate when used for cancer and with anti-seizure drugs.

- **Relationship to the ROOT:** Folic acid is core to the functions of the ROOT, as it concerns cell growth and maintaining immune function.

Vitamin B12

B12 (adenosylcobalamin, cyanocobalamin, methylcobalamin) is a reddish, water-soluble vitamin found in animal foods like meat, eggs, fish, milk, and shellfish. It can also be manufactured by micro-organisms.

- **Functions:** This vitamin is needed to prevent anemia. It plays a vital role in cell growth and DNA synthesis, and acts as a cofactor for fat and carbohydrate metabolism. It also assists in the synthesis of myelin, the fatty sheaths that protect nerves, and hence it aids nerve-cell activity. Together with folic acid and vitamin B6, B12 regulates homocysteine levels. It is required for acetylcholine production in the brain for memory and learning.

- **Intake:** Supplemental doses are encouraged for vegetarians and for those who do not have efficient absorption (particularly protein digestion and absorption).

- **Deficiency:** Lack of B12 can lead to depression, abnormal gait, fatigue, changes in digestion, dizziness, drowsiness, headaches, pernicious anemia, neurological disorders, and skin sensitivity.

- **Overuse:** There are typically no toxic effects from high amounts of B12.

- **Interactions:** High doses of folic acid can mask vitamin B12 deficiency. A number of medications can reduce the absorption or activity of vitamin B12 in the body, including aspirin, antibiotics, and oral contraceptives.

- **Relationship to the ROOT:** Vitamin B12 is connected to the ROOT because of its role in cellular growth and DNA synthesis.

Vitamin C

Vitamin C (ascorbic acid) is a sour, water-soluble compound found in fruits and vegetables, especially citrus fruits.

- **Functions:** This vitamin is most recognized for its antioxidant action (cell protection against free radicals) and its ability to enhance the immune system. It also plays a part in collagen (protein) synthesis and metabolism of amino acids like tyrosine and phenylalanine. Vitamin C is responsible for balancing stress hormones involved in the fight-or-flight response, like norepinephrine and cortisol. The adrenal glands (overseen by the ROOT system) contain one of the highest concentrations of vitamin C in the body.
- **Intake:** Increased amounts of vitamin C, as much as 600–1000 mg per day, have been used to prevent the common cold and for countering high-stress conditions.
- **Deficiency:** Lack of this vitamin can cause scurvy (a disease of deficient collagen that appears as bleeding from all mucosal surfaces, gum bleeding, tooth loss, and skin sores), fatigue, drastic behavioral changes, and gum swelling and bleeding.
- **Overuse:** Excess vitamin C can lead to nausea, vomiting, heartburn, abdominal cramps and gastrointestinal upset, fatigue, headache, and diarrhea. It may lead to the formation of urinary tract stones. Individuals with a history of oxalate kidney stones should monitor their vitamin C intake.
- **Interactions:** Vitamin C may increase the absorption of chromium and iron (from plant sources), and interfere with the absorption of copper. Its use in chemotherapy is controversial.
- **Relationship to the ROOT:** Vitamin C helps to protect the body through its ability to support its defenses via the adrenal glands, production of stress hormones, support of the immune system, and

its antioxidant action. It is typically found in foods that are red—cranberries and other red berries, and even red bell peppers.

Vitamin D

Vitamin D (cholecalciferol) is known as the "sunshine" vitamin. This fat-soluble vitamin, often touted as hormone-like in its action, is created through the interaction of sunlight on the skin or by eating fatty fish, eggs from hens fed with vitamin D, or fortified foods (e.g., milk, yogurt, cereals).

- **Functions:** Vitamin D regulates levels of calcium and phosphorus in the body. It also improves bone health and impacts immune-system activity.

- **Intake:** To prevent vitamin D deficiency and the occurrence of rickets (bone softening and deformity), 200 units (5 mcg) is recommended by the National Academy of Sciences for individuals from birth through fifty years of age; 400 units (10 mcg) is recommended for those older than fifty. However, higher daily doses (800–1000 units) have been recommended for older adults for bone health. A more recent report by renown vitamin D researcher, Dr. Michael Holick, and colleagues suggests that supplemental vitamin D levels should be based on body weight. They found that to achieve an average serum 25(OH)D level >100 nmol/L required vitamin D intakes of 6,000 IU/d for normal Body Mass Index (BMI), 7,000 IU/d for overweight and 8,000 IU/d for obese. Keep in mind that the amount of vitamin D you get naturally through your skin may change throughout the year with varying periods of sunlight. You should alter your dietary supplement requirement accordingly based on your lab and genetic results from a qualified health professional.

- **Deficiency:** Lack of this vitamin can cause rickets, muscle pain, fatigue, possible increased risk for cancer, autoimmune disease, hypertension, and diabetes.

- **Overuse:** Too much vitamin D can result in excess calcium in the body, resulting in weakness, fatigue, headache, nausea, gastrointestinal symptoms, dizziness, and pain in muscle and bone.

- **Interactions:** Vitamin D supplementation may increase intestinal absorption of magnesium. However, it is also important to note that magnesium is required for the metabolism of vitamin D, so taking large doses of vitamin D could induce severe depletion of Mg. Consider concurrent magnesium replenishment if taking higher amounts of vitamin D. If you are unsure as to whether you need magnesium, have your healthcare practitioner measure your blood levels. Exercise caution when using vitamin D in conjunction with drugs or supplements that increase calcium levels in the body.
- **Relationship to the ROOT:** Vitamin D assists in the balance of the primary skeletal mineral, calcium.

Calcium

This chalky, white compound is found in milk products, green vegetables (e.g., kale, broccoli), and canned fish with bones.

- **Functions:** Calcium is found throughout the body, with the majority being present in the bones. However, it is also found in blood, extracellular fluid, and muscle. It is used for a variety of functions, including nerve transmission, muscle contraction, blood vessel activity, and the transport of substances in and out of the cell. It is needed for bone mineralization and used to treat rickets and osteoporosis.
- **Intake:** Calcium is important for preventing osteoporosis in postmenopausal women, where 1000 to 1600 mg elemental calcium has been used. Its absorption can be enhanced when taken together with vitamin D. Calcium supplements at high levels can decrease magnesium, iron, and zinc uptake, however, so it is advisable to take them separately. Several pharmaceuticals interact with calcium supplementation and can lead to changes in calcium levels in the body. If you are taking medications, discuss these potential interactions with your healthcare professional.
- **Deficiency:** Lack of calcium can lead to bone demineralization, PMS, hypertension, stroke, and heart conditions.
- **Overuse:** Excess of calcium can result in hypercalcemia (high blood levels of calcium), kidney stones, arterial calcification, and possible increased risk of prostate cancer.

- **Interactions:** Calcium may interact with antibiotics, diuretics, and thyroid drugs.
- **Relationship to the ROOT:** Calcium helps to support the body through the skeletal framework and muscle fibers.

Copper

This pinkish metal is found in a variety of foods like organ meats, grains, seafood, beef, and cocoa.

- **Functions:** Copper serves as a catalyst in many enzymes (oxidases) in the body. It helps form bone, red blood cells, and proteins like elastin and collagen.
- **Intake:** Patients on hemodialysis may be at higher risk for copper deficiency; supplementation may be beneficial. Copper supplementation (2.5 mg per day) has been used together with calcium, zinc, and manganese for preventing bone loss in postmenopausal women. Individuals who have had gastric bypass surgery may be susceptible to low copper levels. Note that some genetic conditions can lead to toxic copper accumulation in the body, so check with your health-care practitioner before taking copper supplements.
- **Deficiency:** Lack of copper can result in osteoporosis, anemia, baldness, diarrhea, and fatigue.
- **Overuse:** Excess copper can bring on depression, fever, irritability, nausea, joint and muscle pain, and vomiting.
- **Interactions:** Iron, vitamin C, and zinc may decrease copper absorption.
- **Relationship to the ROOT:** Copper plays a role in the intricate interactions among cells, including bone, blood, and muscle, and helps to build protein and support tissue.

Iron

This grayish metal is found abundantly in Earth's crust and foods like meats and vegetables. The highest amounts are found in beef, liver, and lamb; moderate amounts appear in other animal meats like pork and poultry, and in beans.

- **Functions:** Iron assists in the transfer of oxygen and carbon dioxide in the blood through hemoglobin, and in the muscle through myoglobin. It plays a significant role in energy production and utilization.

- **Intake:** For treating anemia due to low iron, 50–100 mg three times daily has been used. Vegetarians and athletes have increased iron needs. However, having too much iron in the body can be toxic for organs like the heart and the liver, especially for those individuals with a genetic susceptibility to storing high amounts of iron called hemochromatosis. Menstruating women who lose blood, and thus iron, and who do not eat iron-rich foods may need to stabilize their ROOT with the anchor of iron.

- **Deficiency:** Iron deficiency can cause anemia, fatigue, cognitive impairment, and hair loss.

- **Overuse:** Excess iron can lead to stomach irritation and pain, diarrhea or constipation, nausea, and vomiting.

- **Interactions:** Calcium, soy protein, and zinc may impair iron absorption. Vitamin C improves absorption of iron from plant sources. Iron supplements may interfere with antibiotics and thyroid medication.

- **Relationship to the ROOT:** Iron supports the ROOT in multiple ways. It is what gives blood its deep red color, and allows the red blood cells to carry oxygen.

Zinc

This bluish-gray metal is found abundantly in Earth's crust and in foods like oysters, animal products, beans, nuts, grains, and seeds.

- **Functions:** Zinc is required for synthesis of protein, DNA, and RNA, prostate gland function, immune-system regulation, wound healing, cell growth, taste and smell, skin health, bone formation, and for the activity of more than 300 enzymes (proteins) in the body.

- **Intake:** Individuals with gastrointestinal disorders that result in nutrient malabsorption (like ulcerative colitis, Crohn's disease, or even diarrhea) can have low zinc due to reduced absorption.

Vegetarians may benefit from zinc supplementation, since animal foods contain more bioavailable zinc than plant foods (plant foods contain compounds called phytates that prevent zinc from being absorbed in the gut). Those who want to facilitate wound healing, as in chronic leg ulcers, may be helped by zinc supplementation. The studies on taking zinc for the common cold reveal mixed results.

- **Deficiency:** Lack of zinc can result in growth retardation, mental lethargy, low sperm count, hair loss, skin dryness and acne, slow wound healing, impaired thyroid function and insulin action, and decreased sense of smell and taste.

- **Overuse:** Too much zinc can cause nausea, vomiting, a metallic taste in the mouth, copper deficiency, gastrointestinal symptoms like diarrhea and stomach upset, and fatigue.

- **Interactions:** Calcium, copper, iron, and fiber may influence zinc absorption. Zinc supplementation may influence the activity of antibiotics.

- **Relationship to the ROOT:** Zinc is vital to the workings of the organs within the ROOT system through its close tie to the functions of protein in the body.

Herbs for Adrenal Support

When it comes to herbs for the ROOT system, there are several classes of plants that are well-known for fortifying the physiological aspects of the ROOT, such as supporting adrenal function (adaptogens), quelling inflammation (botanically based anti-inflammatories), and bolstering immunity (plant-based modulators).

The ROOT is associated with the fear response, which is ideally suited to assist in short-term emergencies. In the body, this response is wired to the functioning of the adrenal glands. Overstimulation of the adrenal glands and excessive stress hormones can drain your energy, as well as cause an inability to think and learn, disturbed sleep patterns, alterations in appetite, and changes in metabolism. Supporting the adrenals with nutritional products is advised for individuals who show these signs of adrenal fatigue. Herbs that act as adaptogens—substances that balance the stress responses, toning down an overactive adrenal response or fortifying a weakened one—can help to heal the endocrine/immune response. Some of these plants include:

Ashwagandha (*Withania somnifera*)
Cordyceps (*Cordyceps sinensis*)
Dang shen (*Codonopsis pilosula*)
Eleuthero (*Eleutherococcus senticosus*)
Ginseng (*Panax ginseng*)
Holy basil (*Ocinum sanctum*)
Licorice (*Glycyrrhiza glabra*)
Reishi mushroom (*Ganoderma lucidum*)
Rhodiola (*Rhodiola rosea*)
Schisandra (*Schisandra chinensis*)

Due to their complexity, it is best to work under a healthcare professional's guidance if you decide to use adaptogenic herbs. Using supplements with adaptogenic properties in conjunction with lifestyle techniques like stress reduction can free you from unecessary fear, stress, and worry.

Anti-Inflammatory Herbs

When the body is inflamed, it exhibits the classical signs of redness, pain, and heat. When it comes to the ROOT system, the joints become painful and swollen, or the skin becomes irritated. In fact, many chronic conditions like obesity, type-2 diabetes, and heart disease are thought to have an underlying inflammation component. Unfortunately, pharmaceuticals that are available to cool the body and fight the inflammatory process also have serious side effects like gastric bleeding and stomach upset. Because of this, natural products that fight inflammation have become even more desirable, although they also carry some precautions regarding their use. Questions to ask yourself if you have an inflamed ROOT system include:

• What makes it so heated?

• Why is its energy erupting into a "volcanic" response?

• How can it best be calmed and cooled?

Here are some herbs that can fight the inflammatory process.

Cat's Claw

The inner bark and roots of this plant (*Uncaria tomentosa*) have been used for their anti-inflammatory, antioxidant, and immune-stimulating effects. Supplementation with cat's claw has relieved knee pain related to physical activity after one week of supplementation. It may also improve symptoms related to rheumatoid arthritis. Taking specific preparations of this plant in extract form at 100–180 mg (60 mg in three divided doses) daily has been shown to be effective for both osteoarthritis and rheumatoid arthritis of the knee. Side effects include headaches, dizziness, and vomiting. However, use of this herb may lead to worsening of motor symptoms in neurological disorders (e.g., Parkinson's disease). Avoid using with immunosuppressants or while taking blood pressure-lowering supplements or drugs. This remedy should not be taken during pregnancy and or by those with an autoimmune disease due to its ability to influence immune function.

Indian Frankincense

This gum resin (*Boswellia serrata*) is used in traditional Ayurvedic medicine, and has been used as an anti-inflammatory and anti-arthritic, as well as to enhance immune function. For arthritic conditions, 333 mg three times daily and 3600 mg daily have been used for osteo- and rheumatoid arthritis, respectively. A study published in 2008 with osteoarthritic individuals indicated that 250 mg of a novel boswellia extract enriched with a specific boswellic acid resulted in improvements in pain and function after just one week of use. Boswellia has also been used for inflammatory gut conditions and asthma. Gastrointestinal effects such as pain, heartburn, nausea, and diarrhea may be experienced while taking the herbal compound. Those with autoimmune disease should be cautious when using this resin due to its immune-modulating effects.

Willow Bark

The willow tree, native to parts of Europe and Asia, has been used since the time of Hippocrates (5th century BC) for its bark, which possesses anti-inflammatory effects. The active compound, salicin, converts into salicylic acid—the same compound found in aspirin. Willow bark works in ways similar to aspirin through its pain-relieving, anti-inflammatory, anti-fever actions. However, like aspirin, its ingestion may also lead to gastrointestinal side effects. Due to its ability to influence blood clotting, this botanical should not be taken in conjunction with anti-coagulant supplements or drugs. This remedy is recommended for short-term use only. For back pain, a willow bark extract containing 120–240 mg salicin can bring relief, with a greater degree of relief experienced at the upper dose. Do not take this herb if you are allergic to salicylates. Side effects include itching and rash.

Herbs for Immune Support

The plants or botanically based actives listed below have been used to bring the immune system into a state of balance, in many cases through stimulation of immunity. A variety of factors can throw the immune system into imbalance, including undue stress, insufficient sleep, poor diet, and inactivity. These plants help heighten the response of the innate immune system. Immune system issues may signal that you need to work on your sense of boundaries and how you discern what is self and what is not self. They may also indicate that you are lacking external support in parts of your life.

These supplements are not recommended for individuals with a hyper-vigilant immune system, as in autoimmune disease. Associated use with immunosuppressant drugs is also not recommended. Since these botanicals are so potent in their immune effects, it may be worthwhile to take them only for short periods of time (approximately four to six weeks), with some time elapsing before the next cycle of supplementation. Finally, note that several of these medicinal plants and plant parts must be taken at the first sign of a cold or flu in order to be effective.

Andrographis

This plant (*Andrographis paniculata*) commonly grows in India and other parts of Asia. The leaves and roots have been used for their antibiotic, anti-allergy, and immune-stimulating properties. It is commonly taken for colds, infections, HIV/AIDS, allergy, and depressed immune function. Side effects include itching, fatigue, headache, diarrhea, nausea, vomiting, heartburn, gastrointestinal discomfort, and anaphylactic reactions. Pregnant women should not use this plant due to potential abortifacient effects. Do not take with supplements or drugs that have anticoagulant, blood-pressure lowering, or immunosuppressive actions. Individuals with autoimmune disease should not take due to potential immune-stimulating effects. A daily dose of 200 mg has been used for preventing the common cold. A specific combination of an andrographis extract and Siberian ginseng has been helpful in treating the common cold and influenza.

Astragalus

This flowering plant (*Astragalus membranaceus*) is typically used for the common cold and upper-respiratory infections, wound healing, injuries, immune-system strengthening, viral infections, chronic fatigue syndrome, and fibromyalgia. Cell studies indicate that it can improve the immune response by stimulating the activity of immune cells. Even though a wide range of doses has been used (1–30 g daily), the typical dose for enhancing immune function is 4–7 g. While well-tolerated overall, doses larger than 28 g daily may cause suppression of the immune system.

Echinacea

Also called "purple coneflower," echinacea (*Echinacea purpurea*) has a long history of use by North American natives for medicinal purposes. Nowadays, echinacea supplementation is advised for preventing the common cold and to assist in recovery from upper-respiratory infections. Although it has been shown to reduce symptoms of the common cold by 10–30 percent in some studies, other studies show no effect at all. Side effects are varied and include nausea, vomiting, allergic reactions (rash, tingling and/ or numb tongue, etc.), bowel-pattern changes, headache, and dizziness. This remedy may interact with the metabolism of several drugs (including caffeine), so be sure to consult a practitioner if you are taking any drugs before taking echinacea. A wide variety of doses have been taken, depending on the preparation (capsules, juice, tea, tincture).

Elderberry

The elderberry fruit (*Sambucus nigra*) is concentrated with numerous plant compounds that function as anti-viral, antioxidant, and immune-stimulating agents. It has been shown to reduce the duration of influenza symptoms by more than 50 percent. A common formulation is elderberry juice syrup. Side effects include weakness, dizziness, numbness, stupor, and allergic reactions (particularly in people with grass pollen allergy).

Lycopene

Lycopene is a red-colored carotenoid from fruits and vegetables like pink grapefruit, watermelon, and tomato. Unlike other carotenoids (e.g., beta-carotene), it does not convert to vitamin A once ingested. In addition to its ability to protect cells as an antioxidant, cell studies indicate that it inhibits cancer-cell proliferation and reduces cardiovascular risk. Supplementation with lycopene may also help reduce the symptoms of exercise-induced asthma. Note that lycopene is a fat-loving carotenoid, so it needs dietary fat or oil to be absorbed.

Sulfates

Sulfates can help support your joints. If you experience joint issues, ask yourself what is preventing you from moving forward or what is keeping you stuck in the past. Then consider utilizing various nutrients like sulfates to rebuild the joint cartilage to prevent further degradation. Do not take sulfates if you have a sulfur allergy or intolerance.

Chondroitin Sulfate

Chondroitin sulfate exists in the body as a part of cartilage structure. These long carbohydrate chains keep cartilage flexible and prevent degeneration by blocking the activity of specific enzymes known to degrade cartilage. Supplemental chondroitin sulfate (typically made from shark cartilage or cow trachea cartilage) at a dose of 200–400 mg two to three times daily, or 1000–1200 mg in a single dose, may be helpful in treating osteoarthritis, although results have been inconsistent.

Often, joint-health supplements will include both glucosamine sulfate and chondroitin sulfate. Effects such as nausea, pain, eyelid swelling, hair loss, and changes in bowel pattern may occur. Do not take together with anticoagulants. Do not take if you have asthma, as it may exacerbate symptoms. Men with prostate cancer or at increased risk of prostate cancer should avoid.

Glucosamine Sulfate

Glucosamine, made from the simple carbohydrate glucose and the amino acid glutamine, is found naturally throughout the body, especially within the joints. In supplement form as glucosamine sulfate, it may help with symptoms of osteoarthritis, including pain relief and better functioning, by rebuilding joint cartilage, although studies indicate mixed results. Side effects include gastrointestinal discomfort and blood-sugar increases.

Glucosamine sulfate is derived from the exoskeletons of shellfish or produced synthetically, so do not take it if you have a shellfish allergy. Do not take together with anticoagulant supplements or drugs, as effects may be enhanced and cause bleeding or bruising. The recommended dose for osteoarthritis is 1500 mg daily or taken in three daily doses (sometimes in combination with chondroitin sulfate, 400 mg three times daily). For knee pain due to previous injury, 2000 mg glucosamine hydrochloride has been shown to be effective.

Methylsulfonylmethane

This sulfur-containing compound, also known as MSM, is found in plants and animals. It is used for a wide array of functions in the body, primarily joint-health issues. Animal studies suggest it may help to decrease joint degradation. Side effects include nausea, gastrointestinal discomfort, headache, fatigue, insomnia, itching, and allergic-type reactions. Common dose range is 500 mg three times daily, up to 3 g twice daily, often used in conjunction with glucosamine sulfate.

CHAPTER 6

THE ORANGE FLOW

One must still have chaos in oneself to be able to give birth to a dancing star.

Friedrich Nietzsche

KEY WORDS FOR THE FLOW: chaos, creativity, duality, emotions, experience, flow, fluidity, movement, orange, partnership, pleasure, relationships, sexuality, water

Our ability to "go with the flow" of our environment resides within the appropriately named FLOW system. In addition to our FLOW representing our flexibility, it holds the sheer pleasure for living and everything that life contains. It is, quite simply, the "fun factor." Without it, we become serious, withered, and desiccated. The FLOW system is represented by the water in our bodies and symbolizes the flux we may experience in our emotional selves. It contains all the materials for creation, like a cosmic dance teeming with chaotic and frenzied emotion, raw creativity, and undulating sensuality. Our FLOW enables us to surrender to chaos and to dive into a state of pure creativity.

E-motions

The very nature of emotion is to be "in motion." All the happiness, sadness, anger, grief, depression, fear, and any combination of these emotions is tied to your FLOW. It is essential to pay attention to your emotions, since they are an expression of your needs. The more you stifle them, the stronger their call to you. Throughout time, society's messages have down-played the expression of emotions, resulting in harm to our health and well-being.

Relationships

The FLOW system represents issues of relationship, both to ourselves and to others. This manifests in a variety of ways, including commitment to relationships, being able to co-create with others, and being considerate and respectful of others. As Sir Arthur Eddington famously said: "We often think that when we have completed our study of one, we know all about two because two is one and one. We forget that we still have to make a study of 'and.'" This focus on the word "and" represents the essence of the FLOW.

The FLOW and Your Body

The FLOW system represents your body's hydration status, particularly as it relates to the colon, which absorbs excess water for the formation of stools, and to the kidneys, which removes bodily toxins via urine. The FLOW also oversees the hydration status of every cell of your being, and the flow of materials in and out of your cell membranes. Because it is responsible for creation and growth in the body, the reproductive system also falls into this system of health. Whereas the ROOT houses the defense strategy of the body, the FLOW comprises the exchange and manifestation of emotions and ideas. Through the conduit of emotions, the FLOW com-municates with other body messengers, like hormones.

The FLOW and Eating

Food and eating represent a functional, survival-based (ROOT) activity, and our bodies incorporate sensory aspects to ensure we eat. When we eat, we eat with all of our senses: sight, touch, taste, smell, and sound. Our physiology and psychology are primed to gain pleasure from our eating experiences. There are specific compounds (peptides) released in the gut when we eat to help our bodies decipher that we are experiencing pleasure from eating. Interestingly, science also tells us that we have taste receptors in the gut—the center of the FLOW system—similar to those found on our tongues. The FLOW system is strongly and tightly woven into our eating experience at a deep, gut, sensory level, similar to that of the ROOT. However, rather than eating for pure survival, we look to food for pleasure with the help of the FLOW.

Researchers from Ohio State University looked at what happened when healthy married couples had a disagreement over a meal. The couples were asked on two separate occasions to eat either a meal high in saturated fat or a meal high in oleic sunflower oil—both with 930 calories and 60 g fat. The researchers measured whether the couples had any pre-existing mood disorders. After the meal, those who were more hostile in their behavior and who already had a history of mood disorders were less efficient in their metabolism. They had greater insulin and triglyceride levels, and a steeper risk in both their inflammatory marker, IL-6, and their glucose. More hostility was also associated with higher levels of the inflammatory TNF-alpha after the meal. No differences were found between the two meal types.

The researchers concluded that, since most people spend about eighteen out of twenty-four hours per day in a post-meal state, and since dining with one's partner is significant, it's worthwhile to be thinking about our mood states. For those people with mood disorders, lack of metabolic efficiency can equate to about an additional 7.6 pounds per year. Maybe it's not so much that your food is changing your metabolism, as that your mood is interacting with your food state and leading to metabolic chaos in your body.

Here are some simple questions you can ask yourself to determine if you are maintaining a balanced FLOW.

Do you allow time to "create" meals?

In our everyday lives, we have become "dashboard diners," consistently eating in our cars during our busy lives. A fair number of us spend a lot of time in our cars, or we are confined to a certain structure of life that stifles our creativity and our ease in preparing meals. Because their lifestyles are so busy, most people do not take the time to indulge in the satisfaction of creating a meal. Several people have admitted to me that they do not enjoy cooking and would rather eat out every night. Julie admitted to me that she dreads the cooking process in any form and does not even find pleasure in eating.

The FLOW system of health gives us the gift of savoring the experience of creating a meal, whether it involves hand-selecting items at the grocery store, designing a visually appealing plate of food, or even inventing new ways of eating through different silverware or painting your own bowl from which to eat. The possibilities of creation through food and eating are truly endless!

Do you create meals with others?

Have everyone participate in the creation of the meal. It's nourishing to your FLOW to create a meal for yourself, but even better if you create a meal for another person, or create a meal with someone. Since the FLOW system aligns to relationships with others, it is good to share your eating occasions. When you share food with another, your senses can become supercharged with delight—eating becomes pleasurable and purposeful. Try inviting someone over to eat and enjoy a meal with you. The more everyone's creativity is invested, the more dynamic the meal experience!

Do you engage your senses when eating?

We often eat mindlessly, and even "senselessly"! When we do, eating becomes an activity to get through, rather than one that invigorates us. Try grounding yourself in the present when you are selecting, preparing, or eating food, so that you can get the most out of your eating experience.

I like to encourage "sensory-rotations"—focusing on one sense a week and applying that to your relationship with food and eating. For instance, if you choose taste as your sense for one week, tune into savoring the multitude of flavors present in a meal or a snack. You may put all of your "taste energy" into one food per day, appreciating its flavor with every bite. If you are a person with a strong affinity for your sense of sight, try tapping into the pleasure of your other senses to get their take on eating. You may discover that sight is your favorite sense for taking a nature walk, but that, when it comes to food, you receive the most richness from your sense of smell. When you select foods at the market, engage all your senses to ensure that you get a whole palette of experience when you sit down to eat!

When you are aware of what you are eating and doing through your senses, you may tend to eat less, because you are in touch with your body and your hunger gauge. By truly being in the moment of the eating experience, you maximize your pleasurable interface and listen to your body. And, when your physiology is happy, your psychology reflects this effect.

Do you play when you eat?

Your creativity may have been stifled as a child, particularly when it came to food and eating. Do you remember hearing "don't play with your food" as a child? Or "eat everything on your plate"—even though that plate was created for you by someone else without the input of your own choice or creativity? For some families, eating can be a serious and somber event. Your FLOW system, however, beckons you to transform this tone into one that is fun and light. Rather than seeing eating as a purely obligatory part of your "daily grind," reflect on how you can turn it into a magical moment of play. When you are eating, sit in the mindset of your childlike self and play with your food in any way that feels right to you.

Try creating food structures and pyramids as part of your meal design using food shapes to dress up the presentation of a meal. One of my favorite tricks is cutting the base of a celery stalk off so it resembles a flower when you look at it from above. I can put this art on a serving dish filled with appetizers. Some clients of mine like to take photos of their meals to capture the aesthetics and play of their food compositions.

Do you eat foods of all colors?

Incorporating foods of all colors into your meals can increase their aesthetic appeal while incorporating a wide range of nutrients. As part of your sensory exploration, the gift of sight can provide so much input. Tune into the colors of foods. Sometimes when I review what someone has eaten, I refrain from commenting on the actual foods; instead, I focus purely on the colors. Did they get their full rainbow spectrum of healthy, whole foods? A variety of colors in the diet signifies that we are eating rich, whole, complex foods.

Let your eyes be tantalized by the colors of food. What catches your eye in the garden or market? When you eat foods, take in and savor the array of colors to nourish your aesthetic eye. Not only are the colors beautiful to observe and take in visually, each of them represents an important physiological function that your body is receiving. Purple compounds, like the anthocyanidins found in grapes, protect the brain and preserve memory function. Orange compounds, like the beta-carotene found in carrots, help maintain vision and a healthy immune system. When you arrange foods on a plate, think about how they fit together in a complementary way. For example, placing diced red pepper or strawberries onto your bed of mixed greens can be very satisfying on both visual and physiological levels.

Do you strive for a balance of tastes?

Traditional forms of medicine like Ayurveda and TCM encourage the use of all flavors in a meal. Research shows that we crave what we do not have in our diets. When on high-protein diets, people crave carbohydrate. When we only eat sweet foods, we crave foods that are savory. It is best to include small amounts of all the flavors in your meals to satisfy your taste buds—both those on your tongue and those in your gut!

Do you express emotions to avoid food cravings?

Experts estimate that 75 percent of overeating is due to emotion. In a stressful, busy society like ours, it becomes difficult to find time to process emotions in a healthy way—for example, through journaling or exercise. As a means of coping with challenging situations, people may feel inclined to distract their emotions by eating. Eating offers a temporary quick-fix solution for having to deal with the flow of a feeling. When people repeatedly engage in emotional eating, they run the risk of letting their unfelt feelings accumulate—a process I call "snowballing." Engaging in emotional eating only adds to the snowball effect, as it can lead to feelings of guilt. This guilt perpetuates the emotional eating cycle. The best approach for your FLOW system is to honor and appropriately express your emotional messages.

Do you observe the symbolism of food cravings?

The foods you crave give you information about your body and your emotions. The fact that you are experiencing a craving lets you know that you have feelings that aren't being felt. In the moment of a craving, do a quick "check-in" with how you are feeling. Are you really craving companionship? Love? Rest and relaxation? Give yourself what you need on a deep level rather than caving in to superficial indulgence. If you are unable to access your emotional state and identify what you really need, look at the qualities and inherent symbolism of the food you are craving.

All foods provide messages about what we need. Because they connect to unfelt emotions, all cravings belong to the FLOW system. Are you craving salty foods like potato chips? Salty cravings connect with your FLOW the most, because, in the body, water follows salt and salt follows water. Craving salty foods may signal that you have a fluid or larger FLOW-system imbalance that requires you to look at the degree of "flow" in your life and how much you are allowing yourself to surrender. Perhaps you find yourself craving sweet foods. Craving these foods may be sending a message that you are lacking sweetness and joy in your own life.

WHAT DO FOOD CRAVINGS SYMBOLIZE?

Each food means different things, depending on the individual. However, there are some basic messages provided by certain foods that we can extract based on the characteristics of that food. When you experience cravings for these foods, ask yourself these questions:

- **Salty**: Where do you need more flow in your life?
- **Crunchy**: What is stressing you? What feels trampled upon and overwhelming?
- **Sweet**: Do you need more joy and fun in your life?
- **Spicy**: Do you crave intensity and living on the edge? Are you afraid of boredom? Are you bored?
- **Sour**: Where do you need to direct your attention? Do you feel scattered?
- **Soft**: What do you need to do to feel comfort? What do you need to do for yourself to feel loved and nurtured?

Do you give your passion purpose?
Cravings may also be linked to insatiable passion that does not have an outlet. When you direct your passion into your life purpose, cravings tend to fizzle out. In another way, you can connect passion to eating by letting it pour into your experience with foods. I find it interesting that people who

are very passionate about life also seem to savor their food to the utmost. When Alan recounts his Saturday evening plans, he delights in describing the minute details of his dinner, including the "zing" of the spices on his tongue from the grilled halibut. He puckers his lips with emphasis when he almost relives eating the blood orange sorbet he made from scratch. When passion infiltrates your life, it can spill over into your experience with foods and eating to make it that much more "juicy" and inviting!

Eating Activities for the FLOW

1. What are your criteria for a healthy relationship with foods and eating? Make an action to become the quality that is first on your list. Write a paragraph on this change.

2. Create a written, positive affirmation to heal your cravings. Write it down on the left side of a piece of paper and write your immediate response to it on the right side of the paper. Do this five times a day for an entire week. Write about any changes in your craving for the food.

3. Set a two-hour artist's date with yourself this week. Involve food and eating. Write about the experience.

4. Make a funny game to help you deal with a food craving. Play is an important ingredient for the FLOW. Consider how you can play with food through games. Create the game and then engage others to bring in the relationship of FLOW.

5. Combine food and creativity in any way you choose, ranging from meal preparation to a unique way to shop at the grocery store. For example, shop only for orange-colored foods. Explore a novel way to grow food, like hydroponics, which uses the water element. Write about your creation and share it with another.

6. Invite someone over for dinner and create a meal together.

7. Pick an emotion that plagues your daily life and journal on how you can better express this emotion throughout your life in a healthy way. How do you "eat" this emotion rather than expressing it? What foods do you gravitate toward when you feel this emotion? What do these foods signify?

8. Keep an extensive log of your food intake and emotions. Have one column for foods eaten and another for emotions felt. At the end of a week, note whether you see any patterns. Do you notice any change in intake when you are feeling more emotional? Are there certain foods you are more or less attracted to during those times?

Foods for Your FLOW

Foods for the FLOW system tend to be flowing in form and high in water and liquid oils. The components of these foods assist us in maintaining easiness, flux, exchange, and pleasure in our lives.

Water

Although it's not a food, water is present in most foods and connects perfectly to the FLOW system. Foods high in water content, or water intake itself, will support your FLOW system. It may seem like common sense, but water is one of the most life-giving substances we can take in. For the most part, we ingest too little water to support our cellular processes. To stay consistently hydrated, it is optimal to sip water throughout the day, rather than gulping it down a glass at a time. A general rule of thumb is to consume half your body weight in ounces of water, with more in the summer or when you have been sweating profusely. When you are properly hydrated, you are better able to "flow" with your emotions and your thoughts, and your overall cellular functioning is better and stronger.

Fats and Oils

Just as protein provides a building block-like structure for the ROOT, fats and oils sculpt a soft framework that helps the body flow through experiences and emotions. Unfortunately, fat has been a misunderstood nutrient for many years. In fact, I have observed this societal metaphor: The denial of fat in our diets is proportional to our inability to experience joy and pleasure. Think back to the advent of low-fat foods in the early 1990s and how, at the same time, we became an increasingly overworked, overburdened society with no time to find pleasure! Rather than focusing on "low-fat" or "no-fat" approaches to eating, the FLOW system craves a balance of healthy fats. The nutritional spotlight needs to swing from an emphasis on the quantity of fat to the quality of fat. The fat found in our current high-sugar, high-fat, processed foods are of low quality. This fat is synthetically derived through a process known as "hydrogenation." The resulting trans fat gives products a longer shelf life, but also helps our bodies to live a shorter life. When we eat this synthetic fat, the body rejects it by exhibiting high "bad" cholesterol and low "good" cholesterol.

In addition to the copious quantities of trans fat in their diets, Americans also eat too many omega-6 fats from vegetable oils like corn and soy. Your body's efforts to offset the balance of fats in your body, especially the omega-3/omega-6 ratio, can put you into a state of hot inflammation. Without the cooling fats from the sea, the omega-3 fats, you can find yourself with any number of inflammatory conditions. One way to balance the ratio of warming and cooling fats is to eat more omega-3 fat from fish, leafy greens, nuts, and seeds. Since these foods are not part of many peoples' diets in appreciable amounts, omega-3 supplements are available.

Fat is unique because it can transform from solid to liquid form depending on temperature. The flexible, flowing, and yet static and stabilizing quality of fat and oil make them the best macronutrients for helping you balance your inner FLOW system. You may think of fat as a gel-like yellow glob, but, in fact, fats are very complex compounds with distinct properties. There are many different families of fat and each one has its own effect in the body. Saturated fatty acids are more solid, rigid fats found primarily in animal products. At a cellular level, these saturated fats can provide some degree of protection to the body, since they are incorporated into the borders around cells. However, too much saturated fat can lead to too much rigidity within the cell, causing chronic diseases.

There are other fats, called unsaturated fatty acids, that are flowing and fluid at room temperature—fats like olive oil, flaxseed oil, and fish oil. These serve a different function in the body. In fact, olive oil is a perfect FLOW food! It's a core food of the Mediterranean diet. Think of how people in the Mediterranean region—Spain, Italy, and Greece—eat. Their meals are very relaxed and easy, not rushed and rigid. Usually, people in these areas of the world like to eat together, in a group of family or friends, with lots of time spent conversing and expressing emotions.

Now let's shift gears. There are some unsaturated, fluid fats that are not made in our bodies. The body can make most fats, including saturated and unsaturated fats, but not the ones in the omega-3 and omega-6 families. This is the reason you need to include these special "essential fatty acids" in your diet. Like all fat, omega-6 and omega-3 fatty acids are needed as building blocks of the walls around the cells called the "cell membrane." Without unsaturated, fluid fat, cells become rigid and do not allow for the easy transport of substances like nutrients and waste products in and out of the cell. With the right balance of saturated and unsaturated fats, cells can release and take in substances, allowing them to function in a healthy manner.

When cells do not have a healthy ratio of unsaturated, omega-6 and omega-3 fats, they cannot function optimally. If you have too few essential fats, you may get dry skin, because the cells in your skin cannot hold water. You may experience hair loss and brittle nails. Your body can take on a rigid quality from the inside out. If you have too much saturated fat and not enough essential, unsaturated fat, you may become more inflamed, developing arthritic conditions or heart disease over a prolonged period.

Healthy oils for the FLOW include:

Almond oil
Butter/ghee (note: avoid if you have a dairy allergy)
Coconut oil
Extra-virgin olive oil
Grapeseed oil
Pumpkin seed oil
Rice bran oil
Sesame oil
Walnut oil

Two fruits, avocados and olives, could also be part of this list due to the high proportion of healthy oils they contain.

Foods that are high in omega-3 essential fatty acids include:

Dark, oily fish, especially salmon, mackerel, tuna
Flaxseed meal
Leafy green vegetables
Walnuts

Nuts and Seeds

The oil in nuts, combined with their high protein content, make them a perfect food for combining grounding (the ROOT system) and flowing (the FLOW system) action. The following nuts are fine choices to support the FLOW system because of the fat they contain:

Almonds
Brazil nuts
Filberts/hazelnuts
Macadamia nuts
Pecans
Pine nuts
Pistachios

Like nuts, some seeds are also rich in healthy fat and so are good for the FLOW. These include:

Flax
Hemp
Poppy
Psyllium
Pumpkin
Sesame
Sunflower

Flaxseed contains oil rich in unsaturated essential fat, as well as compounds called lignans. Lignans act like weak estrogens and are able to compete with estrogen in the body to sit on receptor sites on cells. If the body has too much or too little estrogen, adding plant estrogens like flax to your diet can be beneficial. Because of their ability to influence estrogen activity in the body, these seeds are thought to reduce the risk of breast, prostate, and colon cancers. Check with your health professional about the use of flaxseed meal in your diet and whether it suits your health needs.

Fish and Seafood

The most highly fluid essential fats are commonly found in fish, especially dark, oily fish like salmon. Wild-caught salmon is an almost ideal food for the FLOW, since it is a food that lives in the water and is made of these must-have, fluid fats. And as if that weren't enough, salmon is orange in color—perfect for the FLOW system! Other beneficial fish and seafood sources for the FLOW include:

Anchovies
Catfish
Cod
Crab
Haddock
Halibut
Herring
Lobster
Mackerel
Menhaden
Mussels
Orange roughy
Oyster
Perch
Pollack
Red snapper
Rockfish
Sardines
Scrod
Sea bass
Sole
Squid

Of course, please avoid shellfish or seafood if you are allergic to it.

Note that there can be high levels of methylmercury found in the current fish supply. For those who will not eat fish or who want to limit their intake, essential fatty acids of the omega-6 and omega-3 families can be found in much smaller quantities in leafy green vegetables, seeds (e.g., flaxseed), and nuts. Omega-3 supplements, which are discussed below, are an excellent alternative.

Tropical Fruits

Our FLOW system is the part of us that longs to be soothed with delight, joy, relaxation, and pleasure. Eating fruits grown in tropical areas represents these same qualities. Mangoes, pineapple, papaya, oranges, kiwi, figs, and coconut are superb examples of nourishing tropical fruits for the FLOW.

Orange Foods

As I mentioned already, the color of the FLOW system is orange. A few examples of orange foods include carrots, salmon, yams, orange bell peppers, and oranges. On a nutritional level, most of these orange foods collectively provide beta-carotene (the orange pigment) and other plant carotenoids. These compounds are strong fat-soluble antioxidants that are stored in the fat areas of the body (e.g., under the skin, in the belly) to protect them from damage. Fruits that nourish the FLOW system include:

Apricots
Blood orange
Cantaloupe
Kumquat
Mandarins
Mango
Nectarines
Oranges
Papaya
Passion fruit
Peaches
Persimmons
Tangerines

Vegetables that support your FLOW system include:

Carrots
Orange bell pepper
Pumpkin
Sweet potato
Yam

And, of course, animal products like salmon are ideal for your FLOW.

Supplements for Your FLOW

If your diet isn't supporting your FLOW, you may need to include supplements to keep you flowing on the inside. In this section, I will discuss supplements that can support urinary tract and reproductive health, including oils, vitamins and minerals, and herbs.

Oils

Besides water, oil is essential to keeping you flowing. By their very nature, oils are fluid, and when you ingest them through diet or supplements, you bring that fluidity into your cell membranes. I'll provide more details in this section on various sources for oils and how they can help your FLOW.

Fish Oil

A perfect supplement for the FLOW is fish oil, comprised primarily of the fatty acids known as eicosapentaenoic acid (EPA) and docosahexaenoic acid (DHA). These long-chain omega-3 oils are "body-ready" because they do not have to undergo further conversion in the body. As a result, they can easily be assimilated throughout several tissues, particularly in the brain and eyes. The purity of a fish oil supplement is important to consider, however, since the supply of fish can be tainted with the high levels of methylmercury found in ocean waters. For best results, check to be sure your fish oil supplement does not have a "fishy" taste or smell.

Low amounts of these long-chain omega-3 fish oils in the diet have been shown to be associated with a variety of conditions like heart disease, inflammation, and behavioral disorders. The American Heart Association recommends about 1 g of EPA + DHA per day for individuals with heart disease, and a higher dose (2–4 g) for those with high triglyceride levels. High doses over time may lead to changes in blood clotting and excessive bleeding.

Plant Oil

Borage oil, evening primrose oil, and flaxseed oil are all good sources of healthy omega-3 fats. Flaxseed oil contains high amounts of the omega-3 fat called alpha-linolenic acid (ALA). ALA is the precursor fat to EPA and DHA. If your body needs EPA and DHA, it has to go through an extensive metabolic conversion of ALA, which is not very efficient, since it can be impacted by stress or mineral deficiencies. It has been shown that ALA ingestion does not lead to exactly the same effects as EPA and DHA. However, ALA appears to be important for maintaining cardiovascular health. Flaxseed oil supplementation is an acceptable alternative for those who do not eat fish. Choose organic, cold-pressed sources whenever available. Do not buy oil in a plastic container—only tinted glass or stainless steel—and do not subject it to heat. Like fish oil, high doses of flaxseed oil can lead to changes in blood clotting.

Borage seed oil and evening primrose oil are sometimes used for supplementation, although there is ensuing debate regarding their efficacy. Borage seed oil contains a relatively high level of gamma-linolenic acid (GLA), an omega-6 fat that is anti-inflammatory. Consequently, supplementation with this oil may have anti-inflammatory effects on joints and skin conditions. Likewise, evening primrose oil contains GLA, although in a lower concentration than borage seed oil. Like borage seed oil, it is thought to help with inflammatory conditions like rheumatoid arthritis, eczema, breast pain, and even PMS.

Vitamins and Minerals

Many vitamin and mineral supplements are available to support the FLOW through their effects on hormones, reproductive health, and via their role as fat-soluble antioxidants. Here are a few, along with indications for their use.

Vitamin B6

Vitamin B6 (pyridoxine) supplementation has been shown to reduce PMS symptoms like breast pain, depression, and anxiety. There does not appear to be a dose-response effect, therefore lower doses (50–100 mg) should be used to reduce the risk of side effects. Vitamin B6 supplementation at 100 mg daily was shown to be as effective as the drug bromocriptine without the same degree of side effects. In combination with magnesium (200 mg magnesium oxide), vitamin B6 (50 mg daily) reduced PMS-associated anxiety. See chapter 7 for more details.

Vitamin E

Although most supplemental vitamin E is alpha-tocopherol (d-alpha-tocopherol is the naturally occurring form), the term "vitamin E" actually refers to eight different forms of this fat-soluble vitamin, including alpha-, beta-, gamma- and delta-tocopherols and four tocotrienols. These yellow oils can be found in unrefined vegetable oils, especially wheat germ oil, and in seeds, nuts, and grains.

- **Functions:** Just as vitamin C is a protective water-soluble antioxidant, vitamin E is a lipid-soluble antioxidant, protecting fat in the body from degradation and assisting in the stability and integrity of cell membranes (similar to the role of fat). Each of the individual forms of vitamin E may have a slightly different function and more research is being conducted on their health benefits.

- **Deficiency:** This tends to be rare, but can occur in those who do not absorb fat, or in individuals on a fat-restricted diet. Symptoms include decreased integrity of cell membranes (particularly red blood cells), hemolytic anemia, muscle weakness, neuropathy, infertility, PMS, and increased risk for chronic diseases like cancer, atherosclerosis, and rheumatoid arthritis.

- **Overuse:** Overuse can lead to fatigue, headache, hemorrhage, blurred vision, rash, gastrointestinal distress, and muscle weakness.

- **Interactions:** Do not use in conjunction with supplements or drugs that have anticoagulant activity. High doses of vitamin E may affect the physiological actions of vitamins A and K. Furthermore, vitamin E supplements may increase the metabolism of specific drugs, leading to an amplification of their effects.

- **Relationship to the FLOW:** Vitamin E is a fat-soluble antioxidant and can help prevent oxidation of fat.

Calcium

Like magnesium, calcium is present in a variety of tissues, including the extracellular fluid. Women who eat more calcium-rich foods tend to have reduced PMS symptoms. Calcium supplementation of 1200–1600 mg daily—this may need modification depending on dietary intake—has been recommended as a treatment option for women with PMS. A study in which women with PMS were administered 1000 mg of calcium for three months revealed decreased water retention, pain, and mood disturbances compared to those who took a placebo. It is best to take calcium together with vitamin D. See chapter 5 for more details.

Magnesium

Magnesium is found within the fluid that bathes cells. As a result, it is connected to the transport of substances from cell to cell and therefore to the FLOW system. It is also related to the FLOW through its ability to improve PMS symptoms like fluid retention and mood changes. Daily magnesium doses of 200–360 mg have been found effective. See chapter 8 for more details.

Selenium

Selenium is a metallic substance found in foods like nuts (especially Brazil nuts), crab, liver, fish, poultry, and wheat.

- **Functions:** This mineral prevents the breakdown of fat, especially when combined with vitamin E. It helps to prevent the formation of certain tumors and is needed for the functioning of specific proteins in the body and the production of thyroid hormones.

- **Intake:** Individuals with higher body levels of selenium have been shown to be at reduced risk of cancer. Supplementation with 200 mcg selenium daily decreased cancer incidence by 25 percent.

- **Deficiency:** Lack of this mineral can lead to cancer, high cholesterol, heart disease, exhaustion, growth impairment, and infections.

- **Overuse:** Too much selenium in the system can cause garlic-smelling breath, nausea, vomiting, abdominal pain, fatigue, irritability, hair loss, skin eruptions and/or yellowing, muscle tenderness, and tremors.

- **Interactions:** Vitamin C and zinc may reduce the absorption of selenium. Do not use together with supplements or drugs that have anticoagulant effects.

- **Relationship to the FLOW:** Selenium relates to the FLOW in two ways—by working as a partner with vitamin E to protect the integrity of fat and through its anti-cancer effects.

Urinary Support

The FLOW oversees tissues in the body that regulate water. The primary organs for this activity are the kidneys and urinary tract, which assist the body with removing excess fluid and toxins. Their proper functioning impacts the whole of the system, including the body's level of electrolytes, muscle contraction, nerve transmission, blood pressure, and the pH of body compartments. Problematic symptoms for these organs can arise from the accumulation of micro-organisms within the urinary tract. However, specific nutritional actives can prevent this build-up and keep the tract free of bacteria.

When presented with conditions of the urinary tract, you may find it useful to reflect on the following questions:

- What toxins—emotional, mental, or physical—need to flow through me?
- What emotional excesses am I not willing to release?
- How can I tap into the reservoir of creativity within me?
- Am I confronted with fear?

Two herbal supplements, bearberry and cranberry extract, can provide support for the urinary system.

Bearberry

The bearberry leaf (*Uva ursi*) contains a number of actives, including the bitter agent arbutin, that support its activity as a urinary antiseptic and potentially as a diuretic, making it beneficial for some kidney and bladder conditions. It may also have protective effects on the uterus and may strengthen the heart muscle. This botanical is not recommended for pregnant or lactating women, or for children. It should be taken short-term under the supervision of a qualified health professional. Bearberry can turn urine greenish-brown and cause gastric distress and even liver toxicity in some individuals.

Cranberry Extract

Extracts of the cranberry fruit and cranberry juice are well-known for their ability to prevent bacteria from adhering to the urinary tract. As a result, they may be helpful for urinary tract infections. The cranberry fruit contains a number of plant compounds that acidify the urine. In people with spinal cord injury and bladder dysfunction, supplementation with cranberry extract tablets for one year significantly reduced the incidence of urinary tract infections. Note that cranberry juice and extract may interfere with the metabolism of a number of drugs. Do not take in conjunction with supplements or herbs that have anticoagulant activity (especially warfarin). Avoid cranberry juices that contain added sugars.

Hormone Support

The FLOW is the hub for much hormonal activity because of its connection to reproductive organs. Typically, plant estrogens (called "phytoestrogens") have been used to act as weak estrogens in the body, blocking the strong effects of estrogen, blunting physiological effects related to the binding of estrogen to receptors, or enhancing a weak estrogenic effect in the absence of estrogen itself (as in menopause). Since they work like estrogens, these substances may have other effects in the body—for instance, on bone or neurotransmitters. Because of their estrogen-like actions, individuals with a history of hormone-sensitive cancers should consult their health professionals before taking supplements containing phytoestrogens.

Hormonal imbalances require that we examine our internal balance of feminine and masculine elements. Of course, regardless of whether we are men or women, we all embody the essence of feminine elements—receptivity, warmth, sensitivity, intuition, and grace—and masculine features like assertiveness, independence, authority, analysis, and leadership. If you have hormonal issues that require healing, reflect on the dynamics between your feminine and masculine natures. Are they balanced, or too exaggerated in one direction? Are you able to access either of these characteristics or does one aspect feel more stifled than the other? Examining these aspects may illuminate some aspect of your hormonal imbalance.

Below are herbs that can provide hormonal support and help balance your FLOW.

Black Cohosh

The root of this North American plant (*Cimicifuga racemosa*) has been found to reduce menopausal symptoms, particularly hot flashes. It has also been used traditionally for inducing labor, and preliminary studies suggest it may also favorably impact bone health. Side effects include gastrointestinal upset, rash, headache, weight gain, breast tenderness, and vaginal bleeding. In some cases, liver damage has been reported. Since it may affect the metabolism of a variety of drugs, consult with your healthcare provider before using if you are taking any medications. Women with a family history of breast cancer or with breast cancer should avoid using this, since it is unknown whether it may affect hormone-sensitive cancers. Supplementing with specific black cohosh extracts at 20–40 mg daily has been used in a number of studies to treat menopausal complaints.

Chasteberry Fruit

This fruit (*Vitex agnus-castus*) has been used for an array of hormone-related menstrual complaints, including PMS, breast pain, and painful menses. Individuals taking it should be aware that its influence on hormones and neurotransmitters may result in interactions with drugs that influence these substances. Also, it has been advised that those with hormone-sensitive conditions avoid taking this botanical. Side effects include gastrointestinal complaints, headache, itching, rash, acne, insomnia, and irregular menstrual bleeding. A wide range of doses has been used, and the dose will depend on the unique formulation.

Indole-3-carbinol/diindolylmethane

Indole-3-carbinol (I3C) is a constituent of cruciferous vegetables (e.g., broccoli, Brussels sprouts). When I3C is ingested and exposed to stomach acid, it converts into a number of active metabolites, including diindolylmethane (DIM). Supplementation with I3C (and DIM) has been used to balance hormones, and to prevent various types of cancers, including breast, cervical, and endometrial cancers. It has been shown to be effective in minimizing cervical dysplasia (abnormal cells in the cervix) in a significant percentage of individuals with this abnormality. More clinical research exists for I3C than does for DIM. Although controversial, there is discussion on whether it can promote tumor formation in those who are in the initiation phase of cancer. Side effects include skin rash and, in rare instances, elevations in liver enzymes. The common dose for cervical dysplasia and hormone balance is 200–400 mg daily, with the lower dose working as well as the higher dose in some cases.

Red Clover

The flowers of red clover (*Trifolium pretense*) have been used for a variety of gynecological complaints, including menopausal symptoms, hot flashes, breast pain, and PMS. They contain isoflavones, which have weak estrogenic effects and modulate estrogen activity. Side effects include rash, headache, and nausea. Do not take together with supplements or drugs that have anticoagulant activity. Since it may alter the metabolism of several drugs, consult with your healthcare provider before using this botanical if you are on any medications. Specifically, supplementation may interfere with the metabolism of oral hormones like estrogen and oral contraceptives. Individuals at risk for hormone-sensitive conditions should avoid this supplement. Typical dose for reduction of hot flashes ranges between 40–160 mg daily.

Soy Isoflavones

The isoflavone fraction of soy, particularly genistein, may be helpful for menopausal complaints in some individuals. Daily doses of 35–120 mg have been used for this purpose. Side effects include gastrointestinal upset and headaches. Cautions listed under red clover apply to soy isoflavones. Those who are sensitive or allergic to soy should avoid this supplement.

Gut Support

Just as different fats have to be kept in harmony in the body, so do the different micro-organisms living in our bio-terrain. Seeding the lower gut with healthy bacteria is essential for keeping the gut lining healthy and free of micro-organism overgrowth. These bacteria need to be fed with prebiotics, or special fibers, to keep them active and producing substances that are healthful for the colon. Agents to engage the FLOW system can be helpful for releasing stuck matter and allowing debris to move out.

I have observed that people with lower-gut complaints are in some way linked to the inability to let go—whether that means expanding into their creativity, emotions, or relationships, or releasing any aspects of these things that do not serve them. Utilize the healing element of water through baths, steam rooms, or additional hydration to cause the expansion or release to occur.

Prebiotics

In order to keep the healthy bacteria thriving in your gut, you must feed them. Their food source is prebiotics, or long chains of sugars from fruit and vegetable sources, including asparagus, Jerusalem artichokes, onions, chicory root, and leeks. These foods cannot be broken down by your body's digestive enzymes, but they can be metabolized by bacteria that live in the colon. Two common supplemental sources of prebiotics include fructo-oligosaccharides (FOS) and inulin. Since these both fuel the growth of specific bacteria in the gut, they can work in tandem with probiotic supplementation. A typical daily dose is 4–10 g. Higher doses exceeding 8–10 g daily may result in gas, bloating, and abdominal pain due to the degree of fermentation by intestinal bacteria. Start supplementing very gradually with small amounts, to build up to your gut's tolerance level.

Probiotics

Without adequate amounts of probiotics, the structure of the intestine may degrade, leading to reduced gut immunity and impaired gut movement (peristalsis). Cramping, bloating, loose or constipated stools, and fatigue may result. The two most common micro-organisms with probiotic effects to combat these problems are *Lactobacilli* and *Bifidobacteria*. For keeping a healthy intestinal tract and immune system, try supplementing with one of the many beneficial strains of *Lactobacilli* found in yogurt—*L. acidophilus, L. amylovorus, L. brevis, L. bulgaricus, L. casei, L. crispatus, L. delbrueckii, L. fermentum, L. lactis, L. plantarum, L. reuteri, L. rhamnosus, L. salivarius, L. helveticus, L. paracasei. Bifidobacteria—B. bifidum, B. breve, B. infantis, B. lactis, B. longum*—can also be effective.

Oral therapy with various combinations or doses of these bacteria has been used for acute diarrhea, bacterial overgrowth, atopic dermatitis, immune dysfunction, candidiasis, irritable bowel syndrome (IBS), and ulcerative colitis. When the number of beneficial bacteria outweighs those that are non-beneficial, you can more easily remain in a state of health. If you are taking antibiotics, take your probiotic supplement at least a couple of hours afterward.

Phytonutrients

Plants naturally contain phytonutrients, chemicals that help protect them from germs, fungi, and other threats. These are also called "phytochemicals," both terms derived from the Greek root *phyto* for "plant." Foods like whole grains, nuts, beans, and tea are all rich in phytonutrients, but the most important foods for balancing the FLOW system contain high levels of a compound called beta-carotene (from the carotenoid family).

Beta-carotene

Beta-carotene is an orange pigment that belongs to the family of red/orange/yellow pigments known as carotenoids. It is found concentrated in fruits and vegetables like carrots, sweet potatoes, apricots, peaches, and papaya. Due to its orange color, this carotenoid belongs to the FLOW system. Most of the beta-carotene ingested from foods or supplements converts to vitamin A in the body. The remainder of beta-carotene in the body collects in the skin, adrenals, and corpus luteum. There is no daily recommended dosage for this supplement, but deficiency may be associated with increased damage to cells by free radicals and a weak immune system. Excessive intake can lead to a yellow-orange color of the skin, particularly the palms of the hands and soles of the feet.

Like other antioxidants, beta-carotene in supplemental form has the ability to function in two ways, either as a protective antioxidant or as a potentially harmful pro-oxidant, depending on its environment. Some populations, like smokers and those exposed to high levels of asbestos, have been shown not to benefit from supplementation. My preference is to take all the carotenoids (often labeled as "mixed carotenoids" on a dietary supplement label) together in supplemental form rather than in isolation. Since carotenoids are fat-soluble, it's best to take them in conjunction with dietary fat of some type.

CHAPTER 7

THE YELLOW FIRE

I was always looking outside myself for strength and confidence, but it comes from within. It is there all the time.

Anna Freud

> KEY WORDS FOR THE FIRE: accomplishment, achievement, confidence, ego, fire, goals, inspiration, manifestation, power, presence, self-esteem, transformation, yellow

The FIRE system is our seat of power, which is why I associate it with the color yellow, like the golden color of the sun's rays. Most people living in industrialized countries seem to have an imbalanced FIRE. Through my own research, I have found that up to 80 percent of North Americans and Europeans have a predominant FIRE imbalance. We live in a power-hungry, stress-filled society that is always expecting more and more of us. Our ability to maintain balance in the midst of chaos becomes increasingly difficult when demands and responsibilities begin to pile high. We try to accommodate by saying "yes" instead of "no." Soon after, we feel burdened with life and everyday events become drudgery. Finally, we collapse into a state of exhaustion.

On the whole, your FIRE—and ultimately your entire being—is responding to this current era of excess. We live in an age in which an incredible amount of energy is transferred at faster and faster speeds. For example, we have the Internet, email, and wireless handheld devices so we can be in touch at every moment with the constant stream of information available to us. When we take in too much, however, we may run into difficulty trying to integrate it all.

For example, Sam came to see me complaining of persistent weight gain. Closer examination revealed that he was going through a divorce and had experienced a major job change, and that his daughter was having problems in school. He was barely able to sleep three hours a night. Often, he forgot to eat or ate convenience foods late at night once the kids were in bed. He was experiencing severe internal energy depletion—he was doing nothing in his life to nourish himself. Once he started eating more regularly and eating certain foods, he was better able to concentrate at his new job and began sleeping six hours a night. He began losing weight slowly over the weeks. Four months later, he decided to run a marathon as he had done fifteen years before—he now had the energy for it.

Too much energy given out and an inability to take energy in can cause depletion of physical, mental, and emotional power and lead to chronic disease—particularly diseases centered in the area of the digestive organs. For example, our stomachs can lose their ability to break down and transform foods, which leads to the fermentation of undigested food in the stomach, subsequent acid reflux, and even ulcers.

The FIRE is your energy account. Take a look at your energy flow. At any given moment, you have a certain amount of energy. Many people think of their energy in relation to the past or the future. As a result, they have no energy to live in the present. When you feel drained, you must be careful about how you delegate your internal resources. Are certain external environments leaving you dry? Do other activities give you energy in return?

The FIRE and Your Body

The FIRE system is connected to the organs in the body responsible for transformative processes—in other words, the digestive system, including the esophagus, stomach, pancreas, small intestines, liver, and gallbladder. Your FIRE system is the center of your physical relationship with food. It represents the exchange of food messages and your body's ability to decode that information into signals. The nutrients signal a transformation throughout your body known as metabolism, or the sum of building and breakdown reactions. On a cellular level, this center is linked to your mitochondria, or your cellular powerhouses, whose job it is to extract the raw energy from the starting materials supplied by foods.

On a physical level, people with balanced FIRE systems tend to have robust digestion and metabolism, and they are often of medium build and average weight. These people are the ones who can eat "almost anything" and get away with it. They tend to be able to digest relatively large portions of food in one sitting. Also, people with healthy FIRE systems have energy endurance; they are usually physically and mentally active.

Power, Transformation, and Energy

Food represents energy on many levels, from the physical to the spiritual. All of these energies feed us with the power we need to make our way in the world, whether it's taking a step, uttering a word, or thinking a thought. Our bodies are beautifully equipped with the necessary organs to transform the energy of foods into an energy that we are able to use. The FIRE system is the hub of this transformation. It provides a centralized location for the digestion and absorption of the foods we eat. No other system contains the degree of specialized function for liberating energy that the FIRE system does. The food we eat transforms us. If it carries energy that is nourishing, we become nourished. If it harbors the energy of anger, we take on that anger. Our FIRE is the key for unlocking the messages of food.

Here are a few simple questions you can ask yourself to help you keep your FIRE system burning bright and balanced:

Do you avoid overeating and undereating?
Power signifies a strong current of energy. When we are empowered, our bodies connect with movement to give us direction and focus. When we are able to fuel our bodies appropriately, they can receive the food messages with clarity, helping us to concentrate on the tasks at hand. Many people have lost the ability to recognize if their fuel gauge is on empty or on full. When we overeat, we overwhelm our organs of transformation. Our stomachs take on an uncomfortable feeling, as they are unable to process the

food that has come into them. They remain bloated and acidic, releasing undigested food into the small intestine for future digestion. The small intestine is not always equipped to digest excess food, and may not produce enough enzymes to break down the starches. The liver may not be able to produce enough bile to solubilize the fat we take in.

When you overeat, you impair your body's ability to transform the foods into energy. You may even become drained of energy in the process. Think of any number of large dinners you may have participated in, causing you to feel heavy and lethargic after eating. You can tax your transformative power by excess input of any form, including foods.

On the other hand, not eating enough can lead to a deficit in energy. When you do not eat, you can become low on energy, just as when you overeat. The only difference is that, this time, you are low due to a lack of energy "funds." Under these circumstances, you may also find it difficult to concentrate. The liberation of quick-energy glucose from food helps your brain to function better. When you lack foods, you starve your concentration potential.

It is best to re-train yourself to be in touch with your senses of physical hunger. Note when hunger originates from your gut area, rather than simply "thinking about" being hungry. Is your stomach rumbling? Do you feel an empty pit in that area? If you do, your body is asking you to pay attention and to fill it with fuel, with energy, with power so that you can live a transformative life. This is a signal from your FIRE system that you have put out too much energy and need to take some in to replenish your stores.

When you eat, however, don't saturate your system. Various sources have commented that an optimal intake occurs when you have a sensation of being 80 percent full. My recommendation is that you eat just enough so that, after eating, you can move around comfortably, perhaps taking a light walk. Make sure that you aren't tired after eating, as that can be a sign that you have eaten too much! It may be useful to journal on your food intake and to rate your hunger before and after a meal to see how it compares. Have 1 be "very hungry" and 10 be "painfully full." See what your scores are and whether you are surprised by your ratings. By paying attention to your FIRE system and your hunger times, you will be better suited to deal with the stresses of everyday life.

Can you differentiate between foods that cost and give energy?

Some foods give you optimal energy; some take energy from you. Learn to tell the difference. Have you ever had the experience of eating a small portion of a specific food and feeling as if it wiped you out after eating it? These foods will be different for everyone. Moreover, you may react differently to foods at various times of the day or at random periods of your life. One of my clients commented: "Every time I drank orange juice, it felt like crushed glass in my stomach." Even though most people may enjoy, crave, and need orange juice, some individuals may react to its ingestion. You will usually get a quick, definite reaction from your stomach as to whether or not a certain food suits you.

When you couple eating the foods that cost you energy with overeating, your FIRE system is truly in trouble. Karina relayed how she was in bed for days after having a large lunch of Mexican wheat tortillas. She knew that she didn't do well with wheat, yet she proceeded to eat a number of flour tortillas. Of course, she learned that this combination led to severe imbalance.

On the other hand, some foods may impart a burst of energy. Sue states: "Every time I eat steamed broccoli, I feel full of good, healthy energy. It's like fuel for me to function better."

Do you eat regularly and frequently?

The best strategy for ensuring a steady quantity of energy throughout the day is to eat small meals five to six times daily. When you eat small portions throughout the day, you are able to digest them better. Furthermore, you are able to keep your blood-sugar levels steady, rather than creating sharp blood-sugar peaks and drops that can cause you to feel unstable, lightheaded, and fatigued. Eating regularly ensures that you have the proper amount of fuel to keep you feeling charged throughout your day. That said, small, frequent meals may not be for everyone all the time! Stay in tune with your FIRE to assess your energy inputs and outputs, and you'll know what is right for you.

There are times in the day that you are better able to digest than others. For example, in traditional medicine systems like Ayurveda, noontime is seen as the time that the metabolic fire burns brightest, allowing your body to digest food the best. Conversely, eating late at night is the time that your transformative potential is at its low point. You are unable to process food efficiently in a way that is energizing. It often takes some degree of un-training for people to reverse their pattern of eating heavy dinner meals, but the body does adapt quickly.

Do you know when to have "hot" foods?

The elements of fire and heat go hand-in-hand with the FIRE system. It is through the element of fire that transformation takes place. Cooking food changes its structure, which then changes its digestibility. Eating raw food cools us down and requires our digestive organs to work harder to tear down the strong natural bonds present in plant foods. When we cook food, the structure changes so that it is often easier to digest and absorb. In TCM, raw foods are often not advised for people who overthink (spleen *chi* deficiency).

From a FIRE-system perspective, this idea makes good sense. If you are an over-thinker, you may be depleting your FIRE by putting too much energy into thinking, leaving your digestive tract with little energy to process raw foods. Cooked foods are usually better for people with strained digestion, because their enzymes may not be in large supply or their organs may be less functional. For someone with too much FIRE, having some raw foods may be beneficial, because they can help to dispel some of the pent-up FIRE and have a "cooling effect."

Spicy foods are another type of "hot food." Spices like black pepper speed up the digestion and absorption processes and rev up the FIRE system. They can cause a feeling of heat in the body and lead to sweating. I've observed that, on a more psychological level, people who enjoy spicy food crave intensity and warmth in their lives. Their FIRE systems may not be taking in enough excitement, so they provide this quality through spicy food.

Eating Activities for the FIRE

1. Determine which foods have "power" over you. For example, do you feel drawn to eat certain foods to give you energy? Are there foods you crave? Do some foods make you feel "powerless" after you eat them because they rob you of your vital energy? For example, Jim

struggled with his addiction to caffeine. Throughout the day, he felt pulled to saturate himself with highly caffeinated beverages, starting with several cups of dark coffee in the morning and a few soft drinks in the afternoon. Sometimes he even drank an energy drink in the evening if he had plans to go out. One day, he skipped his morning caffeine routine and became incredibly fatigued and non-productive by early afternoon. He felt like a zombie, completely lifeless and devoid of his drive. Looking deeper within, he came to the realization that caffeine had him in its grip and that much of his energy was determined by his caffeine intake. Rather than allow himself to be fueled by this substance, he decided to take his power back by cutting down his intake, getting to bed earlier, and taking short brisk walks throughout the day to re-energize. He also replaced his sugary snacks with tasty, high-glycemic foods like trail mix. Try this exercise for yourself to explore your power relationship with foods and see if you can come up with solutions to become more power-full without the use of food.

2. Examine the sweetness level in your life. Give it a score from one to ten with ten being most sweet and full of joy. What does your score say? Does your sweetness level need adjustment? List five things—not food!—that you can use to nourish your FIRE and your need for sweetness.

3. Make a list of where your energy is being spent when it comes to foods and eating. Note whether you overeat, don't eat enough, or eat rapidly. Do you spend too much time preparing meals or too little? Do you rush in and out of the grocery store, or do you find yourself in a time warp, getting lost in the multitude of products?

4. Do you eat mindlessly? What do you find yourself doing or even thinking while eating? Observe what brings you into focus and concentration when eating.

5. Practice mindful eating with one item of food daily by doing the following: Hold a raisin in your hands. Close your eyes and feel its texture. Feel the power locked within its wrinkled structure. Imagine the goodness of the sun's rays embedded into every ridge. Now open your eyes and look at it carefully—not in a mode of observation, but

with a loving gaze held by eyes of understanding. See the poetry in this dynamic raisin. Think back to when it was a supple grape and now how fragile it has become. How has it traveled to you and where has it traveled from? How did it connect to the plant of which it was a part? Feel the interconnectedness it embodies and take this in through your eyes. Now put it in your mouth and, before starting to chew, feel the sensation on your tongue. Does it impart any sweetness right away? What does it tell you? See how many times you can chew the single raisin, being mindful of each bite. Before swallowing, think of something you want more of in your life—like balance—and infuse the intention of "balance" into the dissolved matrix of the raisin. Swallow and imagine taking in all the nutritional and intentional goodness of the raisin.

6. Journal a page on how stress jeopardizes your eating. Think of three ways to combat stress and implement one way per week. How do you feel at the end of the month? What in your life has shifted?

Foods for Your FIRE

Foods for the FIRE will supply you with the sustained energy you need to keep your inner flame burning bright. Certain carbohydrates may be able to provide your FIRE with what it needs—everything from quick energy sources like glucose to long-lasting sugar sources like fiber.

Carbohydrate

There are several types of carbohydrate, including simple sugars, complex starches, and fiber. Each type of carbohydrate has a different metabolic effect and each affects your FIRE system in a unique way. Moreover, the quantity and quality of the carbohydrate you ingest can be crucial in balancing your FIRE.

Carbohydrate Quantity

It is important to consider the quantity of carbohydrate relative to other macronutrients in your diet, like protein and fat. There always seems to be a debate about what level of carbohydrate in the diet is best. High-carbohydrate diets, or those exceeding 60 percent of total energy from carbohydrate, are probably excessive for most, whereas extremely low-carbohydrate diets, or those in the range of about 20–30 percent of total energy from carbohydrate, may not feel satisfying to some. You may have to modify the carbohydrate level of your diet depending on where you need your inner fuel gauge to be.

The Glycemic Index

There are different types of carbohydrate, from simple sugars to complex starches, each providing specific types and amounts of energy. If you need a slow release of energy to accommodate a consistent output, you are best served by carbohydrates that slowly release sugar (glucose) into the bloodstream. These carbohydrates are often referred to as having a "low glycemic index." Often, but not always, low-glycemic-index carbohydrates are referred to as complex carbohydrates. For example, lentils represent both a low-glycemic-index and a complex carbohydrate. On the other hand, an apple may be considered a quick energy source, since it consists of simple sugars. However, the sugar it contains is primarily fructose, which has a low glycemic impact.

To understand the glycemic index better, think of the sugar entering your bloodstream as water coming out of a faucet. If you turn the faucet on all the way so that the water streams out rapidly, you fill up the sink quickly. In much the same way, when you eat foods that have a high glycemic index, the simple sugars from the food quickly stream into the blood and your blood sugar spikes. On the other hand, when you eat low-glycemic-index foods, you release sugar into the bloodstream slowly—the faucet dribbles out a little water every couple of seconds. Foods that have a low glycemic index—grains, beans, and vegetables—are nourishing to your FIRE system. Foods that have a high glycemic index are less helpful, providing only a "quick-fix." Some high-energy foods that deplete your FIRE are:

Fruit juices with added sugar
High-sugar desserts like cakes, cookies, donuts, ice cream, candies
Processed breakfast cereals
Starchy snack foods like crackers, potato chips, tortilla chips

Starchy vegetables like corn and white potatoes
Processed grain products (e.g., bagels, muffins, sliced bread)
White rice

Science has shown that eating low-glycemic-index foods results in a panorama of health benefits, including improved body weight, balanced blood lipids, and stable blood sugar and insulin, as well as better appetite control. Rather than have your hunger cues be out of control, or even having your appetite control you, low-glycemic-index foods help you keep a better rein on your hunger and give you energy!

One word of caution, however. Not all low-glycemic foods are healthy and not all high-glycemic foods are unhealthy. For example, ice cream is a low-glycemic food and watermelon can have a high-glycemic impact. So use the glycemic index as just one decision-making factor in assessing which foods are right for your FIRE.

Fiber

Fiber refers to the part of a plant that is not able to be digested. On a basic level, there are two types of fiber: soluble and insoluble. Insoluble fibers are the non-digestible carbohydrates that go through your digestive tract relatively unchanged. They are usually referred to as being "broom-like," in that their structure moves through the long tunnel of the intestines, carrying other bulk through with it. These fibers are for moving digested food and other secretions through the intestinal tract. They are found in the outer skin of fruits, vegetables, grains, nuts, and beans, suggesting that they serve as protection for these whole foods.

The other type of fiber, called soluble fiber, helps sustain your energy. These fibers are found underneath the insoluble fiber sheath of plants. For example, an apple contains insoluble fiber in the red skin, and soluble fiber in the whitish flesh of the fruit. Soluble fibers have a structure that enables them to swell in the presence of fluid. They become viscous and gel-like and are able to form a matrix to trap particles like sugars so they can be released slowly into the bloodstream. This extended release helps you harness your energy input by stabilizing blood sugar.

Unfortunately, most people don't eat enough fiber of any type! It is important to eat high-fiber foods when you are engaged in strong mental or physical activity—competing at a sport or even working at the office. These foods prevent drastic fluctuations of glucose in the blood—sharply spiking and then plummeting within a short period of time. High-fiber foods stabilize the release of glucose into the blood stream for a constant energy level.

Foods that are good sources of insoluble fiber include:

Fruits
Nuts and seeds
Vegetables (carrots, cucumbers, zucchini)
Wheat bran
Whole-grain foods

Foods that are good sources of soluble fiber include:

Flaxseed meal
Fruit and fruit juices (tomato, plum, berries)
Legumes (dried peas, lentils)
Psyllium seed husk
Vegetables
Whole grains (oats, rye, barley) Note: Avoid gluten-containing grains like barley, rye, oat, wheat, and spelt, if you have celiac disease or gluten intolerance.

Quick-Release Sugars and Sweeteners

Foods that release quick, rapid bursts of simple sugars—cookies, soft drinks, and candy—can block or imbalance your energy supply. These foods tend to be processed and refined, not whole and complex. For example, orange juice reacts differently in the body compared with eating an orange. The juice, made from the collection of simple sugars from more than one orange, is high in those sugars and gives a quick burst of energy to the body. Eating an orange, however, results in a slow release of the natural sugars from the matrix of the fruit into the body.

Foods high in simple sugars cause a burst of energy to enter the body rapidly without a compensatory constant output. In fact, much of the body's digestive and metabolic resources are utilized to balance the body after the ingestion of these foods. Have you ever noticed how tired you feel an hour after having a sugary snack? Initially, the burst of energy may feel energizing, but as your body processes the sugars quickly, you are left in a "sugarless" state. You feel used up and tired. You may even get into a cycle of reaching for another sugary snack to inflate your energy once again. If the pattern continues, you may throw off your careful metabolic balance and set yourself up for conditions like obesity, metabolic syndrome, and subsequent development of diabetes.

SUGAR ADDICTION

Most of us are addicted to sugars. When you eat high-intensity artificial sweeteners and processed sweeteners like high-fructose corn syrup, your body's baseline for sweetness reaches an unnatural state. After a certain time, it is difficult to find anything like natural sugars or fruits that are satisfying because of the high "sweetness expectation" you have created. The real question is: Why are you craving such high-intensity sweetness? What sweetness are you missing in your life? What is out of balance? As you may recognize, people who are burdened with stress and responsibilities burn up the energy in their FIRE. Their natural reaction is to look for sweetness in their foods to give them the temporary sensation of energy and delight. However, by doing so, they are setting themselves up for further drains on their energy.

Of course, high-intensity sweeteners are disguised in many forms. Here are the names of some natural and artificial sweeteners to look for on labels:

Aspartame
Acesulfame potassium
Brown sugar
Confectioner's sugar
Corn sugar
Corn syrup
Dextrose
Evaporated cane juice
Glucose

High-fructose corn syrup
Honey
Maltose
Molasses
Powdered sugar
Raw sugar
Saccharin
Sucralose (Splenda™)
Sucrose
Turbinado sugar

Sweeteners that are more balanced (and have a low glycemic index) are fruit juice concentrate and stevia. Personally, I prefer honey and maple syrup, since these two sweeteners also contain other healing compounds.

Jane's case is a perfect example of someone trapped by high-intensity sweeteners. She started her morning with sweetened cold cereal and a white-flour bagel with honey. On her way to work, she stopped for an iced latté. By ten in the morning, she already felt her energy dragging and could not focus on her work. So she ate some candy to help her pick up her pace, which helped initially, but she quickly found herself back to feeling exhausted. By mid-afternoon, she was so sleepy that she had at least one soft drink to give her some caffeine. It is no wonder that she came home in the evening so exhausted that she couldn't make dinner or go to the gym to exercise. However, once Jane eliminated all sources of processed sweeteners in her diet, she realized that her sugar cravings had stopped entirely within ten days. Her tastebuds started to get used to the sweetness of whole fruit and of healthy, natural sweeteners like honey. Her fatigue dissipated and she was able to function better in her job. Changing her diet helped her to focus on adding more sweetness in her life through an evening class on watercolor painting. Her FIRE was brought back into balance!

Whole Grains

If you are used to consuming processed, fiber-poor grains on a regular basis—for instance, ready-to-eat cereals and white bagels—chances are you are depleting your FIRE. In fact, refined grains seem to be a trigger food for many people, since they can behave like quick-release sugars in the body. We may become easily addicted to their quick energy if it is not balanced by whole, unrefined grains. Whole grains like steel-cut (not instant) oatmeal, cooked pearled barley, bulgur, and buckwheat are superb sources of quality carbohydrate like fiber and starches. I like to recommend that clients choose gluten-free grains whenever possible, like brown rice, millet, quinoa, and amaranth.

Gluten is a protein found in grains like wheat, barley, rye, spelt, and, in some cases, oats (through contamination with other grains). Some people are unable to digest gluten and, as a result, cannot eat most grains. In the past five to seven years, an increased number of gluten-free processed products have been put on the market. This increase could reflect a higher number of individuals developing gluten sensitivity, or it may indicate a heightened awareness that gluten intolerance exists at high numbers. It is worthwhile to note, however, that many of these processed, gluten-free products tend to be higher in sugar. Generally, products that have a particular ingredient removed—fat, sugar, or salt—tend to have increased amounts of another ingredient. People following a gluten-free regimen and eating store-bought products may find themselves eating greater quantities of refined sugar, which, as we discussed, is not ideal for a FIRE system that requires healing.

Some people exhibit increased body weight when they have too many grains in their diet. Many times, they are eating too many refined grains, spiking their blood-sugar levels and causing their appetite to run out of control. However, some people can't even eat whole grains. Their digestive tracts are not able to process grains for any number of reasons. I recommend that these people refrain from eating grains entirely. Once they get their lives into balance, they may be better able to handle grains in their diet and feel less inclination to "overdo" them.

As a society, we have become so used to eating grains. We start off with pancakes for breakfast, eat a sandwich for lunch, and have spaghetti for dinner. By doing so, we inundate our bodies with too much refined energy. Couple that with all the external demands we must face, and you can see that we can easily overwork our poor FIRE systems I have observed that my clients who are addicted to grains tend to lead busy lives that are full of worry and stress. By bringing your life into balance and focusing on the needs of your FIRE, you will be less prone to binge on grains.

Legumes

Legumes aren't for everyone, but for those who can tolerate them well, they provide a balanced source of both protein and fibrous carbohydrate. Here are some legumes you may want to consider including in your diet:

Adzuki beans
Black beans
Black-eyed beans
Butter beans
Cannelloni beans
Fat-free refried beans
Fava beans
Garbanzo (chickpea) beans (includes hummus)
Green beans
Kidney beans
Lentils (orange, green, brown)
Lima beans
Mung beans
Navy beans
Pinto beans
Soybeans (could be dry roasted or fresh edamame, but make sure
   they are organic!)
White beans

Starchy Vegetables

Starchy vegetables like corn and potatoes are high in glycemic impact, yet, in their organically grown forms, they can be eaten in small amounts in combination with other foods. Other starchy vegetables that have healthy phytonutrients include:

Acorn squash
Corn (cornmeal)
Parsnip
Potato (gold, purple, red, sweet)
Pumpkin
Taro

Winter squash
Yams
Yellow summer squash
Yucca

Low-Glycemic Foods

Low-glycemic vegetables and fruits include:

Apples
Berries
Broccoli
Cauliflower
Cherries
Dark green leafy vegetables (spinach, kale, dandelion, collard, etc.)
Grapefruit
Green peas
Pear
Tomatoes

Low-glycemic legumes include:

Adzuki beans
Black beans
Black-eyed beans
Butter beans
Cannelloni beans
Fat-free refried beans
Fava beans
Garbanzo (chickpea) beans (includes hummus)
Green beans
Kidney beans
Lentils (orange, green, brown)
Lima beans
Mung beans
Navy beans
Pinto beans

Soybeans (could be dry roasted or fresh edamame, but make sure
they are organic!)
White beans

Low-glycemic nuts and whole grains that support your FIRE include:

Barley (note: contains gluten)
High-fiber wheat tortilla (note: contains gluten)
Nuts and nut butters (unsweetened)
Oatmeal (whole rolled oats, steel cut oats; look for gluten-free
options)

Yellow Foods

While many yellow foods—those that are highly processed and have a
high glycemic index—should be avoided, there are some yellow, tan, or
golden-colored foods that can help your FIRE to burn brightly. For
instance, lemon juice or fresh lemon in water are excellent tonics for the
liver. Refrain from eating corn and corn-derived products if you are allergic to corn. Yellow-colored fruits that support your FIRE system include:

Bananas
Grapefruit
Lemons
Pineapple
Plantains

Vegetables and legumes that help balance this critical system include:

Corn (whole organic)
Garbanzo beans
Ginger
Lentils
Yellow bell pepper
Yellow split peas
Yellow string beans
Yellow summer squash
Yukon gold potatoes

And finally, grains that help your FIRE burn bright include:

Amaranth
Brown rice
Corn meal
Millet
Polenta
Quinoa
Whole grain breads
Whole grain cereals

Supplements for Your FIRE

Digestion is a problem for many people. There are many dietary issues for the FIRE system, such as gluten intolerance, grain and legume intolerance and/or allergy, and excessive sweeteners of all types. In fact, it almost seems that, for the FIRE, it's more about removing foods than it is adding them. In this section, I discuss which supplements to include to help you get your FIRE system back to the zen-like balance it craves!

Soluble Fiber

For most of us, our FIRE systems are on constant overdrive—we are continually burning the candle at both ends. To help maintain your energy reserves, choose carbohydrate sources of the slow and complex variety, like soluble fiber, for a long, continued supply of energy. In supplement form, bulk soluble powders made from psyllium seed, guar gum, and fruit pectin are available. They work to clear the intestines of toxins and soften the stool. The action of these soluble fibers comes from their capacity to swell and become gummy when eaten (which is why they need to be consumed quickly after mixing with water). Including soluble fiber with a meal helps to slow the release of sugar into the blood, assisting in the balance of blood sugar. In the lower part of the gut, soluble fiber can be fermented by bacteria, creating nutrients like short-chain fatty acids that keep the colon healthy. Make sure to rotate your dietary supplemental fiber sources, as some people with digestive issues can easily develop sensitivities to them.

Vitamins and Minerals

Many vitamins and minerals can serve as support for the FIRE system. For instance, the entire B vitamin complex—eight water-soluble vitamins including B1 (thiamin), B2 (riboflavin), B3 (niacin), B5 (pantothenic acid), B6 (pyridoxine), B7 (biotin), B9 (folate), and B12 (cyanocobalamin)—is essential to FIRE health. Although each of these have functions separate from the others, when treated as a complex, they all contribute to an efficient FIRE, assisting in energy production from carbohydrate, protein, and fat.

Vitamin B1

Vitamin B1, or thiamin, is a water-soluble vitamin found in whole grains, legumes, meats (particularly liver), egg yolks, vegetables, and fruit.

- **Functions:** This is an important nutrient for carbohydrate metabolism. Eating large amounts of carbohydrate increases the need for thiamin. It is also essential for nervous system activity, brain function, and cognition.

- **Deficiency:** People consuming a diet high in refined carbohydrate or high in alcohol are susceptible to thiamin deficiency. A deficiency manifests as a condition referred to as "beriberi," or neurological symptoms like nerve pain, exaggerated reflexes, and diminished sensation in hands and arms ("dry beriberi"). It also may present as cardiovascular symptoms like rapid heart rate, enlarged heart, and breathing difficulties ("wet beriberi"). Deficiency may also cause brain abnormalities.

- **Overuse:** Side effects are relatively uncommon.

- **Interactions:** Consumption of large amounts of coffee and tea can convert thiamin into a form that cannot be used by the body. This reaction can be prevented with adequate intake of vitamin C or by ingesting sufficient thiamin. Raw fish and shellfish contain an enzyme that degrades thiamin. Cooking inactivates this enzyme.

- **Relationship to the FIRE:** Thiamin is an essential vitamin required for carbohydrate metabolism.

Vitamin B2

This water-soluble vitamin, also known as riboflavin, is found in cheese, egg yolks, fish, legumes, meats, and milk.

- **Functions:** Riboflavin assists in metabolism of carbohydrate, fat, and protein through its role in cellular respiration, or harnessing energy from macronutrients. It is also needed for red blood cell formation, antibody production, and metabolism of tryptophan, and may be useful in carpal tunnel syndrome.

- **Deficiency:** Deficiency can result in cracks or sores at the corners of the mouth, dermatitis, hair loss, light sensitivity, decreased mental response, and eye disorders. Strenuous exercise may increase the body's need for riboflavin.

- **Overuse:** No direct toxic effects are known in humans, but very high doses may lead to cataract formation, retinal diseases, and diarrhea. Can also cause a yellow-orange discoloration of urine.

- **Interactions:** B2 may improve iron utilization.

- **Relationship to the FIRE**: Like its sister B vitamins, riboflavin helps in metabolic pathways to maintain a steady flux of energy exchange.

Vitamin B3

Also known as niacin, niacinamide, and nicotinic acid, vitamin B3 is a water-soluble vitamin found in beef liver, brewer's yeast, vegetables, dairy products, whole grains, red fish (tuna, salmon), coffee, and tea.

- **Functions:** Niacin is used for the metabolism of carbohydrate, fat, and protein (oxidation-reduction reactions) and for the synthesis of the body's energy currency, ATP. It reduces cholesterol in its niacin/ nicotinic acid form only and does not work with niacinamide. Niacin can be synthesized from the amino acid tryptophan if sufficient vitamin B6, riboflavin, and iron are available.

- **Deficiency:** Severe niacin deficiency results in a condition called "pellagra," or a constellation of symptoms including a thick, scaly rash, a bright tongue, vomiting, diarrhea, depression, headache, memory loss, and, ultimately, death if left untreated.

- **Overuse:** Too much nicotinic acid can result in a facial flush, some-times experienced with a tingling sensation, after ingestion. Nia-cinamide ingestion does not cause facial flushing. Ingestion of high amounts of either one (nicotinic acid or niacinamide) can lead to nausea and vomiting, and liver damage. It may decrease the action of insulin, resulting in an impairment of the body's ability to use glucose.

- **Interactions:** Avoid alcohol intake when taking vitamin B3 sup-plements. People who have frequent attacks of gout should refrain from supplementation. Exercise caution if taking with statins due to potential heightened risk of muscle soreness (myopathy).

- **Relationship to the FIRE:** All vitamins contribute to energy pro-duction; however, this vitamin is particularly involved in metabo-lism. Since vitamin B3 is directly involved in metabolism reactions and is required for making ATP, it has an integral role in the FIRE. It is truly a "powerhouse" energy supplement for your physical body.

Vitamin B5

This water-soluble vitamin, also known as pantothenic acid or calcium pantothenate, is found throughout the food supply. Its name is derived from the Greek word *pantothen*, meaning "from everywhere."

- **Functions:** B5 is essential for the metabolism of carbohydrate, pro-tein, and fat, and for the function of the adrenal gland and produc-tion of adrenal hormones.

- **Deficiency:** Low B5 is relatively rare, perhaps due to the ubiquity of pantothenic acid in foods. It can manifest as fatigue, headache, nausea, tingling in hands and feet, muscle weakness in legs, gastroin-testinal complaints, and increased susceptibility to infections.

- **Overuse:** Effects from overuse are not typical, but can result in diarrhea.

- **Relationship to the FIRE:** Pantothenic acid is needed for the metabolism of all the macronutrients.

Vitamin B6

This water-soluble vitamin, also known as pyridoxine, is found in a wide variety of foods, including cereal grains, beans, animal foods like meat and eggs, and some fruits and vegetables.

- **Functions:** As part of the entire B vitamin family, vitamin B6 plays a role in metabolism of macronutrients, especially protein. On its own, it is integral to forming hemoglobin, the protein in the blood that carries oxygen. It also keeps the heart healthy through its reduction of the damaging amino acid product homocysteine. It assists in the synthesis and metabolism of neurotransmitters like serotonin and dopamine.

- **Deficiency:** Lack of B6 can lead to dermatitis, sore tongue (glossitis), depression, confusion, convulsions, and anemia.

- **Overuse:** Doses over 100 mg daily are not advised due to the potential to cause changes in nerve function. Other indications of overuse include nausea, vomiting, loss of appetite, abdominal pain, and headache.

- **Interactions:** B6 may interfere with the effects of some drugs, particularly those that impact the brain and nervous system.

- **Relationship to the FIRE:** Like the other B vitamins, vitamin B6 assists with metabolism.

Vitamin B7

Vitamin B7, also known as biotin, is a water-soluble vitamin found in brewer's yeast, cooked eggs, meat, milk, and whole grains.

- **Functions:** Biotin regulates the metabolism of carbohydrate, protein, and fat. It affects cell growth, fatty-acid production, and B-vitamin utilization, and contributes to healthy hair, skin, and nails.

- **Deficiency:** Lack of biotin can cause anemia, depression, hair loss, scaly rash, lethargy, impaired utilization of glucose leading to increased blood sugar, muscle pain, soreness of tongue, and nausea. Deficiency may result from consumption of raw egg white for an extended period (weeks to years). Cooking egg whites denatures the protein that prevents the absorption of dietary biotin.

- **Overuse:** Not known to be toxic.
- **Relationship to the FIRE:** Through its effects on metabolism, biotin helps the FIRE system stay healthy.

Vitamin B12

In addition to its many roles associated with the ROOT, vitamin B12 is required in the metabolism of fat and carbohydrate under the direction of the FIRE system. The presence of a particular protein (intrinsic factor) in the stomach is needed for its absorption into the body. Therefore, a healthy functioning stomach (and FIRE system) will be essential for vitamin B12's functions in the realm of the ROOT system. See chapter 5 for details.

Chromium

This trace element appears in a wide variety of foods, including grains, seafood, beef, and dairy products like cheese.

- **Functions:** Chromium plays a pivotal role in metabolism of macro-nutrients, particularly carbohydrate, and is used for improving the body's ability to dispose of glucose (sugar). Supplementation is often advocated in diabetes and in conditions associated with blood-sugar imbalance like hypoglycemia, decreased energy, and polycystic ovary disease.
- **Intake:** The recommendation for type-2 diabetes is 200–1000 mcg in divided doses throughout the day. Newer research shows a blunting of food intake and cravings in overweight women taking 1000 mcg of chromium versus placebo.
- **Deficiency:** Deficiency may occur with stress, malnutrition, and pregnancy. Diabetics may have lower body chromium levels. Symptoms include poor glucose control, nerve dysfunction, and weight loss.
- **Overuse:** Too much chromium can lead to weight gain, cognitive and nerve dysfunction, headaches, sleep disturbances, mood changes, vomiting, and kidney damage.
- **Interactions:** Chromium competes with iron and zinc for absorption and transport, so take them separately. If you take chromium

supplements together with insulin, hypoglycemia may result. Do not take thyroid medication (e.g., synthroid) at the same time as a chromium supplement.

- **Relationship to the FIRE:** Chromium lends a hand to the FIRE system by allowing energy in the form of glucose to be efficiently delivered and received by the whole body, especially in the liver and muscle.

Blood-Sugar Support

When glucose balance is thrown off in the body, it is a sign that there is imbalance in your FIRE. The body's inability to use glucose effectively spills over into other systems, too. For example, extended periods of dysglycemia (abnormal levels of glucose in the blood) will lead to changes in the blood vessels and the circulation of blood, altered appetite, difficulty in concentration and focus, and nervous-system dysfunction like nerve pain in the outer extremities. Regulating blood glucose levels is essential to maintaining the balance of the entire body.

When blood-sugar balance is an issue, ask yourself these questions:

- Where am I squandering my resources?
- Why am I not finding sweetness in my life?
- What are some things I can do to make life more enjoyable?
- What opinions, beliefs, and thoughts can I release to make life more enjoyable?

Alpha-Lipoic Acid

This is a potent antioxidant that aids in carbohydrate metabolism and has been used to improve tissue sensitivity to insulin in diabetics at 600–1200 mg daily. It helps to regenerate antioxidants like vitamins C and E and is used extensively to reduce symptoms of diabetic nerve pain (see chapter 11). Nausea and skin rash have been reported with its use. There may be additive effects when taken with other hypoglycemic agents.

American Ginseng

The ginseng root (*Panax quinquefolius*) is an ancient tonic to restore energy and combat fatigue. It helps reduce the amount of stress hormones that congest the FIRE-system organs, thereby helping hormones like insulin to work more effectively. Taking 3 g before a meal can lower blood glucose in diabetics. Do not confuse American ginseng with Siberian or *panax* (Asian) ginseng. Side effects include gastrointestinal complaints, insomnia, and agitation (especially in schizophrenics). Ginseng may increase the action of supplements or drugs with hypoglycemic activity. Do not take together with monoamine oxidase inhibitors or with warfarin. Since some ginseng extracts have estrogenic effects, those with a history of or with active hormone-sensitive cancers should consult their health professional before using.

Bitter Melon/Bitter Gourd

Bitter melon (*Momordica charantia*) is a vegetable commonly eaten in Asian countries that can lower blood glucose. A number of actives in bitter melon that influence insulin action have been identified. It may be taken as a fresh juice (very bitter) at 50–100 ml daily, as a dry powder (3–15 g daily), or as a standardized extract (100–200 mg three times daily). Tolerance has been suggested to be acceptable at 3 g per day (1 g three times daily). Excessive intake can lead to diarrhea, and gastrointestinal upset and pain. Note that taking bitter melon with other herbs or supplements that reduce blood sugar can have an additive effect and cause hypoglycemia. Not recommended for use in pregnancy.

Cinnamon

Although there are conflicting data, cinnamon (*Cassia cinnamon*) may impact glucose and insulin levels favorably. In diabetes, 1–6 g daily (1 tsp. = 4.75 g) has been used. Large amounts may be toxic to the liver. Do not use in conjunction with supplements or drugs that have hypoglycemic or hepatotoxic effects.

Fenugreek

Fenugreek (*Trigonella foenum-graecum*) seeds, possibly due to their soluble fiber content, have been shown to decrease blood-sugar levels in diabetes at 15 g daily (soaked in water) or in the form of an extract (1 g daily). Fat in the blood may also be reduced with fenugreek supplementation, although further research is necessary. Side effects include gastrointestinal complaints, hypoglycemia in large doses, and allergic reactions. Exercise caution when using together with supplements or drugs that have anti-coagulant or hypoglycemic actions. Do not use in pregnancy or lactation. Not to be taken by children.

Gymnema

This woody shrub (*Gymnema sylvestre*) is native to India and Africa. Its leaf has been used for thousands of years in India to treat "honey urine" (diabetes). A 400 mg extract of gymnema taken daily by diabetics has reduced blood sugar. It is thought that it works by decreasing the uptake of sugar in the intestines and also by stimulating the beta cells that produce insulin in the pancreas. Use caution if taking together with blood-sugar lowering supplements or drugs.

Digestive Support

Over time, with aging or stress, the ability of your digestive system to extract energy from foods may become impaired. The breakdown of foods starts in the mouth with the production of amylase to degrade starch. If you do not chew your foods adequately and give careful attention to what you put into your mouth, it may be more difficult to digest and assimilate these substances in the body. Various supplements, like digestive enzymes, can be used to assist in the process. If you continue to ingest foods without being able to digest them in the mouth, stomach, and intestines, you can become inadequately nourished to deal with your daily events, adding to the stress in your FIRE system. Moreover, the undigested food makes its way farther through your intestine and, in the presence of a leaky gut, may result in large food particles being taken up by the systemic circulation (seen by the body as "invaders"), ultimately causing an immune reaction.

One of the first organs of transformation within the FIRE system is the stomach. With too much incoming energy that cannot be processed effectively, the stomach may become overheated, inflamed, acidic, and unable to digest. Potent yellow botanicals like turmeric and ginger can provide the stomach with the healing compounds it needs to cool down and move energy through the body.

When digestive disorders arise, ask yourself this question: What am I not able to assimilate or "digest"?

Digestive Enzymes

Commercial enzyme preparations made from animal or fungal sources are available to assist in the breakdown of the three main macronutrients: protein (proteases), carbohydrate (amylases), and fat (lipases). These three types of enzymes are often combined in supplement preparations. Since they work directly on ingested food, they should be taken with the meal. Do not drink large amounts of water during mealtimes as this may dilute the enzyme concentration and impair their activity.

Ginger Root

The yellowish ginger root (*Zingiber officinale*) has traditionally been used to treat stomach upset, nausea, vomiting, and morning sickness. Although it has a reputation as being protective to the stomach, it can cause stomach distress like heartburn, abdominal pain, or diarrhea if taken in large amounts. Ginger has also been used to reduce inflammation, thin the blood, and lower cholesterol. Due to its blood-thinning properties, it is not recommended for those who take anticoagulants. Likewise, individuals who have gallstones should avoid it, since it has stimulating effects on bile secretion. One of ginger's most common applications is for morning sickness: 250 mg ginger four times daily or 500 mg twice daily has been used for this indication. For healthy stomach movement, 1000–1200 mg ginger has been studied. Extended use during pregnancy is not advised.

Hydrochloric Acid

Lack of significant stomach acid to digest dietary protein commonly occurs with aging. Supplemental hydrochloric acid (for example, in the form of betaine hydrochloric acid) can be taken with meals to assist the stomach in this process. See chapter 5 for more details.

Turmeric

Turmeric (*Curcuma longa*), commonly used as a seasoning and as a constituent of curry powder, has been shown to exhibit strong antioxidant and anti-inflammatory properties. Taking 500 mg four times daily or 600 mg five times daily has been shown to reduce dyspepsia symptoms. The major actives are the curcuminoids. Side effects may include nausea and diarrhea. Use caution if taking together with anticoagulant supplements or drugs.

Liver Support

The liver is very consistent with the workings of your inner FIRE: it filters out what the body does not need through its concentration of enzymes. This process occurs through two sequential steps. The first is the conversion of toxins into water-soluble compounds; the second is the addition of a chemical group like a sulfur-containing compound to assist in their release from the body. For this reason, your ability to clear the metabolic clutter from within comes from the liver.

In addition to being one of the major organs of detoxification, the liver is the central site for processing fat. After eating, the fat from the meal travels through the systemic circulation in a protein-containing compound. The last stop is typically the liver. Too many fatty foods, highly processed foods full of sugar, or overconsumption of alcohol may cause congestion in the liver. Various nutritional approaches can assist this precious organ in its ability to detoxify body poisons and dispose of fat in the body.

Liver issues like fat accumulation, inflammation, or toxicity may require examining the efficient function and energetics of the liver. What is preventing you from action? What toxin, either from the environment or from within (e.g., emotions, thought patterns) is causing you to become stuck and inflamed?

Choline

Choline used to be considered a B vitamin until it was discovered that it could be produced in the liver. Dietary sources include egg yolks, liver, meats, nuts, and wheat germ. Choline assists in gallbladder regulation and prevents liver dysfunction. Choline deficiency can lead to fatty liver (hepatic steatosis), most likely due to its role in fat and cholesterol metabolism. Choline helps reduce levels of homocysteine, a harmful amino acid that has been correlated with heart disease, and is a building block for acetylcholine, the neurotransmitter responsible for memory and mood. In choline deficiency, brain function and memory are impaired. Finally, choline is required for the transmission of nerve impulses from the brain through the central nervous system. Side effects of choline supplementation include profuse sweating, fishy body odor, gastrointestinal complaints, and vomiting.

Dandelion Root

The bright yellow dandelion plant (*Taraxacum officinale*) has traditionally been used for liver complaints, as a diuretic, and to stimulate appetite. It may have some impact on the digestive process through its ability to increase bile production. Dandelion should not be taken in conjunction with prescription diuretics, or by those with biliary tract obstruction or gallstones. It may also alter how certain drugs are metabolized, so check with your healthcare professional if you are taking medications. In some individuals, it may cause allergic reactions.

Milk Thistle

The seeds of the milk thistle (*Silybum marianum*) contain the potent active silymarin, which is particularly effective for treating liver disorders. It prevents toxin infiltration into the liver cells, stimulates new liver-cell growth, and may possess anti-inflammatory, immune-enhancing properties that are particularly beneficial in liver conditions. It may help decrease insulin resistance, reduce dyspepsia, and protect against kidney damage. It is generally well tolerated, but allergic reactions and gastrointestinal effects like laxation may be experienced. Milk thistle supplements may alter the metabolism of specific drugs like warfarin and diazepam. The plant extract (not necessarily the seed) may have estrogenic effects; therefore, individuals with hormone-sensitive conditions should avoid it. Individuals with an iron storage disease (hemachromatosis) should avoid taking milk thistle. Different preparations and doses have been used: for hepatic cirrhosis, 420 mg of a milk thistle extract containing 70–80 percent silymarin; for chronic active hepatitis, a formulation containing 240 mg silybin (administered twice daily).

Metabolism Support

The bulk of B vitamins are instrumental in helping to fuel the metabolic reactions for carbohydrate, protein, and fat, typically by playing a role in core processes like cellular respiration or in oxidation-reduction reactions. Since the FIRE system is directly linked to the element of fire, try to apply this connection symbolically with that of the "metabolic fire." Ask yourself how you burn fuel (nutrients) for energy. If your metabolism is slow, what in your life needs igniting or catalytic action?

Green Tea Extract

Green tea extracts rich in the polyphenol epigallocatechin gallate (EGCG) can increase fat and calorie burning along with suppressing appetite. The individual constituents in green tea, including caffeine and catechins, may be responsible for these effects. Side effects include gastrointestinal complaints, agitation, dizziness, insomnia, tremors, confusion, and potentially liver toxicity (particularly when taking a specific ethanolic extract of green tea). Exercise caution when taking in conjunction with supplements or drugs that have anticoagulant activity. Additive effects may occur when taken with other caffeine-containing products. Green tea reduces the absorption of iron from plant sources and may decrease the activity of folic acid. Do not use together with supplements or drugs that have stimulatory effects on the central nervous system. A recent study showed that a supplement containing a green tea extract composed of 890 mg polyphenols and about 366 mg of EGCG led to increased fat-burn16ing and improved insulin sensitivity in healthy humans compared with a placebo. Similarly, overweight men taking 300 mg of EGCG for just two days led to more fat-burning than when they were taking a placebo.

L-Carnitine

L-carnitine, a compound related to the structure of amino acids that is derived from animal foods, assists in transporting long-chain fats into the mitochondria so they can be burned for energy. The human body can make L-carnitine if sufficient iron, thiamin, vitamin B6, vitamin C, lysine, and methionine are present. L-carnitine can convert in the body to acetyl-L-carnitine when needed (see chapter 11). Low levels in the body can lead to mental confusion, heart pain, muscle weakness, and obesity. Supplementation may be useful in conditions where there is impaired fat metabolism. Conditions involving fatigue, like chronic fatigue syndrome and autoimmune diseases, may most benefit. Side effects include gastrointestinal disturbances, fishy body odor, and seizures. This supplement interacts with thyroid hormone and supplements or drugs that have anticoagulant properties. Dose for combating fatigue related to a clinical condition is 2 g daily.

CHAPTER 8

THE GREEN LOVE

It is only with the heart that one can see rightly; what is essential is invisible to the eye.

Antoine de Saint-Exupéry

> KEY WORDS FOR THE LOVE: breath, compassion, depth, devotion, emotional wisdom, empathy, forgiveness, giving, gratitude, green, joy, kindness, love, loyalty, receiving

The heart takes on a special meaning for many. References to the heart and love are used in our everyday language. The word "love" also takes on a variety of meanings, from romantic love to platonic love to familial love. In fact, "love" has become a ubiquitous word—"I loved that movie!" "I love going on vacation." If you take a moment to reflect, it may seem that every event in your life is a call to love, whether it's an angry outburst, a teary goodbye, or bitter silence. At the root of every dysfunction is our unfulfilled need to be loved deeply. When we do not feel loved, we act out to get the attention we desire.

The LOVE system encompasses the physical heart, which sits deep in the center of the body. It takes on a mystical quality for most of us for good reasons. There is now some research that may indicate why we are such "heart-struck" beings. Our hearts may, in fact, be the seat of our intelligence. Dr. Rollin McCraty has reported that the magnetic field of the heart is "around 5000 times stronger than that produced by the brain" and can be "measured several feet away from the body." Have you ever walked into a meeting and felt a sudden shot of anxiety running through your chest before anyone has uttered a word? Or, before shaking hands with someone, have you gotten an immediate impression of them as you enter the room? Your heart allows you to "feel" situations without the need for any words or actions. Most people believe that it's the brain that gives us our sense of perception. However, emerging research is revealing that the heart's ability has been grossly underestimated.

Studies have shown that compassion is a healing force that practitioners can employ with patients. Dr. Larry Dossey commented: "The majority of healing studies suggests that a healing effect is real and mediated by compassion and empathy." Love melts resentment, anger, and bitterness, and turns them into a beautiful landscape of forgiveness and joy. Since love is such a big deal for us, it is no wonder that most of our health issues are related to the heart. Heart disease continues to be the number one killer of both men and women. When we block our ability to forgive, we block our arteries, our blood vessels. We get high cholesterol. We eventually get heart attacks. Through connecting with the love inside us, we soften our hearts and keep the circulation of our blood moving healthily.

The messages our society sends out hint at an open, giving heart as being a healthy thing, which it can be. When we hear phrases like "open-hearted," "big-hearted," "warm-hearted," we may think of an individual who possesses beneficial qualities like kindness, generosity, and lovingness. However, the LOVE system is not a one-way street. As you may imagine, repeated giving unbalanced by receiving can lead to "compassion fatigue."

The LOVE and Your Body

As the name suggests, the LOVE system is associated primarily with the heart and lungs. The heart and lungs share an intimate relationship, as they work together for the single goal of pumping oxygen via the blood to the rest of the body. Peripheral to the heart and lungs, the LOVE governs the breasts, shoulders, armpits, arms, wrists, and hands. The arms are essentially an extension of the heart, as they are the tools needed for the important healing activity of touch and reaching out to others. Finally, the blood vessel network throughout the body is connected to the LOVE, as it is the means by which blood and oxygen can be delivered throughout the body.

The LOVE and Eating

For the ROOT, FLOW, and FIRE systems, food and eating serve the physical body—its instinct for survival, its need for pleasure, and its requirement for transformation and energy. For the LOVE and other systems, food and eating lose some of this physical emphasis, and take on a more symbolic significance.

There is a high level of ritual that corresponds with eating. Some religions and spiritual practices include a prayer, grace, or offering of gratitude at the beginning of a meal. It may begin at the hunt for an animal, giving thanks to the animal for sharing its life and energy with the tribe, or even at the point of picking fruits and vegetables for a meal. In several cultures, food is used as a way to show love. Dating couples may celebrate by going out to have a meal at a restaurant. Mothers bake cookies for their children and cook meals for their families. Grandmothers like to serve a treat when you come over for a visit. Essentially, if we care about others, we feel the need to share food with them, whether preparing it for them, serving it to them, or even eating along with them. We extend the love we have through the conduit of food.

Also, it is through the act of eating that we show that we value and love the bodies we have. If we didn't care for ourselves, we would stop eating altogether (unless the act of starvation was linked to a cause). Some traditions have used the phrase: "Your body is your temple." Indeed, loving ourselves implies providing ourselves with constant, quality nourishment.

When you enter into an eating experience with an open, loving heart, you magnify the healing effects of foods compared to eating from a place of non-love. The greatest nourishment you can ever take in is that of love and compassion. Love infuses every morsel of food you ingest. Without it, you starve your heart and, ultimately, your soul.

Who we love is connected to what and how we eat. You may have heard the phrases: "You are who you love" and "You are what you eat." Both contain inherent wisdom. When you love someone, you develop a heartfelt connection with that person, like an invisible cord of energy that runs between the two of you. The level of bonding can be so deep that the feelings felt by each one may be shared by the other, either knowingly or not. As a result, we may end up eating similarly to those we love.

This concept was demonstrated in a large published study in the *New England Journal of Medicine*. Drs. Christakis and Fowler demonstrated that patterns of body-weight gain were directly connected to our social networks. In other words, the greater the connection an individual has with obese friends and family, even if miles apart, the larger the influence on his or her developing obesity. So, if your emotionally close friend is obese, there is a higher chance of you becoming obese.

In a similar way, research has shown that children's eating behaviors are influenced by their parents, particularly girls patterning their mothers. One of the best things parents can do for their children is to ensure that they are setting a consistent example of healthy eating.

Here are a few simple questions you can ask yourself to determine if you have established and are maintaining healthy eating patterns that can support the LOVE system.

Do you eat and serve food with love and gratitude?

Have you ever had a meal made with love, or had all of the parts of the meal lovingly created, prepared, and served to you? If you have, you know what a treat it is and how it feeds your body along with your spirit. People who buy organic food claim that it tastes better than conventionally grown food, even when they do not know which one is which. There certainly is an element of "love" that appears to go into organic gardening. And when you select an organic food, you actively tap into the love that has been grown into the food from the sun, stars, moon, sky, farmer, harvester, and grocer.

If you haven't experienced it, or even if you have, try to feel love in every cell of your being while you prepare food. Start by feeling love and compassion coming from the magnificent lotus of your heart with every slice, simmer, and sauté, and see whether you notice the difference throughout your body and in your energy level. Chances are that, if you are preparing and eating food with love, you will feel a warm kindness radiate through you while you eat and after eating, due to the opening of your heart as it responds to the love in the food.

ONE BOWL

Author Don Gerrard has published a book on the concept of eating from one bowl for every meal. When you concentrate your love and intention into your eating vessel, he claims, food and eating take on an elevated meaning. You become more aware of what you are putting into your bowl and how that nurtures you. Many people also choose to use the same utensil. For example, I choose to eat with a small teaspoon with a rose on the handle. Doing so helps me to take in and savor small bites, and the rose is a reminder of the beauty and love associated with foods.

Do you share meals with others?

When we share love, we receive more back—the love in our hearts grows exponentially. In a similar way, sharing meals with others feeds our hearts. Cathy describes how she dreaded eating because she ate alone. When I recommended that she invite others over to eat every Sunday afternoon, eating took on a whole new meaning and feeling for her. She looked forward to Sunday and inviting new guests and trying new recipes. The process of invitation to others opened her heart. Food became a passion for her. Eventually, she was invited as a guest to other homes and was welcomed to eat in their presence.

Eating in a communal setting is so important for us as human beings. We are social by nature. Our lives in a spiritual sense are truly about giving and receiving love. When we build walls around us, we close off our hearts. Eating with others can create so much joy, especially when the meals are prepared together. Eating with others, just like praying with others, intensifies the energy received from the experience.

Eating Activities for the LOVE

1. Have a serving of green vegetables (1 cup of fresh salad greens or ½ cup of steamed broccoli or Brussels sprouts) at least once daily. Note whether you have any resistance or whether you welcome this action. How do you feel when you eat them?

2. Create a prayer of gratitude and grace to say before your meals.

3. Sing while you prepare food. Sound helps the lungs to open, and since the lungs are opening wide, the heart is also affected.

4. Focus on your breath while eating and synchronize your breath to your rhythm of eating. Breathe deeply and chew thoroughly. What messages of the heart are you unlocking with every bite?

5. Make a meal with love and share it with someone you love. How does it taste? Does it taste different than a meal made without love?

6. Put heart stickers all over your food packaging and containers (e.g., water bottle) to remind yourself to love yourself and your food.

7. Eat one raw food or leafy green-containing meal daily for one week. Note whether you feel any different at the end of the week.

8. Do you use food to show love? Have others used food to show love to you? How has this been beneficial or detrimental? What are alternate ways to show love?

Foods for Your LOVE

The ROOT, FLOW, and FIRE systems revolve around the macronutrient universe of protein, fat, and carbohydrate. In fact, most nutrition texts focus on these powerhouses of the dietary world. We eat several grams of each of them every day, and the sheer quantity of macronutrients makes up the bulk of our eating. However, there are some nutrients that never get to take center stage, yet they can be as important. These are called phytochemicals or phytonutrients (*phyto* is the Greek root for "plant"). These tiny pigments and compounds impart color and protection to plants, and bring health benefits to people. There are several thousand of them in our food supply and their effects have significant potential. Overall, with its strong connection to nature and plants, the LOVE system is represented by vegetables and their respective *phyto* compounds: phytochemicals, phytoestrogens, phytosterols.

Vegetables

Before diving into the teeny-tiny territory of "phytos," it is worthwhile to start with the physically large, visible food influences on the LOVE: vegetables.

Cruciferous Vegetables

Cruciferous vegetables, like broccoli, cauliflower, and Brussels sprouts, are especially balancing for the LOVE system. The cruciferous vegetables share a common stinky, sulfur smell, indicating that they are effective at guarding the body from toxins. Sulfur-containing compounds like sulforaphane act as detoxification agents in the body. Observe your reactions to green vegetables, as it may provide a small mirror of what is happening within your LOVE system on a symbolic level. I have worked with several people who simply will not eat green vegetables. Jessica states: "My parents would steam broccoli and the smell was so awful! It would fill the house, making me feel sick." Others have commented the opposite. Jeff reports: "One of the reasons I enjoy green vegetables is because I feel closer to the earth; I like their earthy flavor." It is very common to hear how good and vibrant people feel when they eat green vegetables.

Cruciferous vegetables that help to nourish the LOVE system include:

Arugula
Bok choy
Broccoflower
Broccoli
Brussels sprouts
Cabbage (green, red)
Cauliflower
Chinese cabbage
Collard greens
Daikon
Horseradish
Kale
Mustard greens
Napa cabbage

Wasabi
Watercress

Leafy Greens

If you take time to notice the physical structure of leafy greens, you will see that their leaves are full of circulating life. The tiny web-like imprint that is embedded into the leaf vaguely resembles the circulatory system. These airy, raw, and open leaves provide us with the freshness of nature that we need to feel. Fresh leafy salad greens contain nutrients like folate and vitamin K to keep our hearts protected. Not only is folate important for the reproduction and maintenance of cells; it is one of the protectors against high levels of a compound called homocysteine, which can injure blood vessels. Vitamin K, another building block of greens, helps oversee the flow of blood. Without adequate vitamin K, blood does not clot appropriately, something that is necessary to prevent us from bleeding if there is an injury or accident.

Finally, leafy salad greens like romaine, red leaf, butterhead (bibb), escarole, iceberg, and spinach are perfect to eat during lunch time, when the sun is at its peak—which also coincides with the time that our internal "metabolic fire" burns brightest. These greens keep us calm, cool, and collected in the midst of external and internal "fire" that can be very damaging to our tender hearts.

Leafy greens that help to nourish the LOVE system include:

Arugula
Bok choy
Chard (rainbow, red)
Collard greens
Dandelion
Kale
Mixed greens
Mustard greens
Romaine
Spinach
Sprouts (of all types)
Watercress

Fruits and Legumes

Fruits that support the LOVE system include:

Avocado
Green grapes
Honeydew melon
Kiwi
Pear

Legumes that contribute to the balance of the LOVE system include:

Green beans
Green Northern beans
Green split peas
Soybeans (edamame)

Phytochemicals

Researchers have slowly been uncovering the population of phytochemicals within our foods. Walsh and other researchers suggest that there are up to 10,000 of these found in the layers of fruits, vegetables, whole grains, and legumes. And to think that we may have limited ourselves to focusing on only the three nutritional musketeers: protein, fat, and carbohydrate!

Many times, these phytochemicals are what give plants their color. For example, lycopene is the phytochemical that makes a tomato red; beta-carotene is what makes carrots orange. These and other potent phytochemicals are what is missing from the infamous, modern-day brown/yellow/white-foods diet.

Phytochemicals are not just about making plants look pretty by adding color, however. They serve particular physiological functions within the body. Without them, we miss out on important health benefits. Foods that are grown organically produce different phytochemicals to make them hearty in a stressful environment. Eating plant foods, particularly those of the rainbowed, organic, unprocessed variety, brings our hearts back into happy mode.

Chlorophyll

An example of an incredibly power-full, heart-loving phytochemical is chlorophyll, which could perhaps be named "king of the phytochemicals." Foods high in chlorophyll, like spirulina, wheat grass, and chlorella, are nourishing for the heart through their positive health effects on the blood and circulation. Chlorophyll is the basic building block of all plants and is responsible for transforming light into energy in plant structures. In our structures, chlorophyll provides the necessary nutritional element to bind toxins so that they can be excreted. As a result, the blood remains pure and free of contaminants. Moreover, foods high in chlorophyll are cooling and anti-inflammatory, probably due to their antioxidant action.

Foods rich in chlorophyll include:

Alfalfa grass
Barley grass
Chlorella
Green vegetables
Spirulina
Wheat grass

Phytoestrogens

Since the LOVE system embraces the breast region, it is essential to take in plant compounds that support the breasts and hormone activity related to the breasts, particularly in women. Certain foods are rich in plant compounds that resemble estrogen, although they have only a fraction of the activity of estrogen. These compounds are often referred to as *phytoestrogens*, or plant estrogens.

In some individuals, phytoestrogens may prevent some of the potential damage created by estrogen binding to receptor sites in the breast by binding in their place. As a result, the breast tissue is protected from the possible negative effects of estrogen, especially in the case of estrogen-related breast cancers. There is, however, some debate about whether these foods should be consumed by individuals who have had estrogen-sensitive cancers. Consult your health professional about whether or not phytoestrogenic foods may be beneficial for you.

Foods high in phytoestrogens include:

Black beans (dried or fresh)
Flaxseed meal
Garbanzo beans (dried or fresh)
Lentils (dried or fresh)
Oat bran
Pinto beans (dried or fresh)
Soybeans (dried or fresh)
Vegetables
White beans (dried or fresh)
Whole grain breads and cereals

Phytosterols

Phytosterols (plant sterols) are a particular type of phytochemical that look similar to cholesterol, without the negative effects. Phytosterols are found naturally in virtually all plant foods, including nuts, seeds, whole grains, and vegetables. Their primary role is to block cholesterol absorption in the body and to keep cell membranes healthy.

Supplements for Your LOVE

Getting vegetables into your diet may be challenging; however, it is one of the most worthwhile steps you can make for your health, especially your LOVE system. Even though you may be doing your best, you may need to take specific supplements to heal your cardiovascular and respiratory function. In this section, I give you what you need to get started.

Macronutrient Supplements

Protein and its amino acid components can provide important support for your LOVE system. L-arginine and organic soy are primary elements for balancing cardiovascular and heart function.

L-Arginine

This amino acid from animal foods may be helpful in cardiovascular conditions like coronary heart failure, angina (chest pain), and high blood pressure, as well as for blood vessel impairments like erectile dysfunction. L-arginine is converted into a compound (nitric oxide) that allows the blood vessels to expand. Side effects include abdominal pain and bloating, diarrhea, and gout. Do not combine with supplements or drugs that lower blood pressure or that open blood vessels. For congestive heart failure, 6–20 g has been given in three divided doses per day. For high blood pressure, 6 g daily has been used therapeutically (in combination with other nutrients).

Organic, Non-GMO Soy Protein

High-quality soy protein derived from edamame is a nourishing protein source for the heart, mainly due to its ability to lower blood fat and blood pressure and prevent cardiovascular disease. For lowering blood fat, 20–50 g of soy protein daily is recommended.

Soy protein is unique because it contains all the amino acids necessary to support growth; therefore, it is one of the few vegetable proteins that can be used efficiently by the body. In addition to being a nutritionally complete protein, it contains an array of other nutritional actives for the heart: phytoestrogens (isoflavones, lignans), phytosterols, and minerals.

Besides its effects on blood fat, soy protein has the potential to influence other LOVE-system organs, including the breasts. Population studies with Asian women indicate that a diet high in soy foods results in a reduced risk for breast cancer. However, studies in the North American population are lacking. More research is needed to understand the role of soy in breast cancer. Women with breast cancer or a history of breast cancer should reduce or avoid soy intake due to the lack of knowledge regarding its effects.

Soy protein, particularly due to the content of isoflavones, may reduce hot flashes and the overall severity of menopausal symptoms. Other benefits of eating soy may include increased bone-mineral density and improved markers of bone turnover in women. Side effects include gastrointestinal upset like changes in bowel pattern (constipation, diarrhea), bloating, and nausea. Individuals who are allergic to soy should avoid it. For those with iodine deficiency, high intake of soy may inhibit thyroid hormone synthesis. It has the potential to interact with monoamine oxidase inhibitors, oral estrogens, tamoxifen, and anticoagulant drugs.

Vitamins and Minerals

In this section, I address some of the key vitamins and minerals that can help you to establish more balance in your LOVE system, including better blood-fat levels, and improved clotting and heart rhythm.

Vitamin B3

Vitamin B3 is also commonly known as niacin. One of its primary uses is reducing high blood fats like LDL-cholesterol (the "bad" cholesterol) and triglycerides, and increasing HDL-cholesterol (the "good" cholesterol). Since high doses of niacin are usually needed for effects on cholesterol (1200–3000 mg per day), it is found not only in dietary supplement form, but also as a prescription drug. Niacin is often taken in combination with statins (prescription drugs to lower cholesterol); however, this should only be done under the supervision of a qualified healthcare professional, as there is a potential for a worsening of the side effects of statins. The main side effect with high doses of niacin (not niacinamide) is flushing in the face, neck, and chest. See chapter 7 for more details.

Vitamin B6

Vitamin B6 (100–200 mg daily) works together with folic acid to reduce levels of the blood-vessel-damaging compound homocysteine by about one-third. See chapters 5 and 7 for more details.

Vitamin K

This fat-soluble vitamin is found primarily in leafy green vegetables like broccoli and spinach, and in vegetable oil like soybean oil. It is also known as phylloquinone, or Vitamin K1.

- **Functions:** Vitamin K is required for normal blood clotting and for a healthy bone structure. Supplementation of 5 mg vitamin K for two to four years resulted in fewer fractures in postmenopausal women with low bone-mineral density.
- **Deficiency:** Lack of vitamin K can cause excessive bleeding due to abnormal blood clotting (for example: nosebleeds, bleeding gums, heavy menstrual bleeding). Taking certain medications like antibiotics may result in vitamin K deficiency.

- **Overuse:** There is no known toxicity with high doses.

- **Interactions:** Supplementation with both coenzyme Q10 and vitamin K may lead to additive effects (increased blood clotting). Vitamin E reduces the absorption of vitamin K and can alter its activity in the body. Vitamin K may reduce the activity of anti-coagulant medications like warfarin (Coumadin).

- **Relationship to the LOVE:** Vitamin K plays an essential role in the normal coagulation of blood, as in the case of a wound or injury where the skin is broken and bleeds.

Iodine

Iodine supplementation (80 mcg of molecular iodine per kg body weight) has been used for fibrocystic breast disease. The breast tissue concentrates iodine to a greater extent than the thyroid gland. Women with breast cancer have lower iodine levels in their breast tissue compared to women without cancer or women with benign fibroadenomas. Populations that have greater iodine intakes, as in Japan, have lower breast cancer incidence relative to those populations with lower iodine intakes. The relationship between dietary iodine and iodine supplementation and breast cancer continues to be investigated. See chapter 9 for more details.

Magnesium

This silver-white alkaline metal is found within the Earth's crust and in a wide variety of foods like legumes, grains, vegetables, seeds, nuts, dairy products, meats, and chocolate.

- **Functions:** Magnesium is used for the activity of hundreds of enzymes in the body. The skeleton is a depository of magnesium, but it can also be found in the fluid in which cells are bathed, facilitating reactions. Magnesium supplements are often taken for cardiovascular disease. Doses of 450–1000 mg daily have been used for high blood pressure.

- **Deficiency:** Lack of magnesium can lead to confusion, insomnia, gastrointestinal issues, rapid heartbeat, diabetes, cardiovascular issues, chronic pain, and fatigue.

- **Overuse:** Excess of magnesium can cause diarrhea, nausea, vomiting, muscle weakness, and heart irregularities.

- **Interactions:** Supplementation with high doses of calcium or zinc can decrease magnesium absorption, so it is best to take them separately. Several medications can interact with magnesium supplements and also alter magnesium levels in the body. Check with your healthcare practitioner if you are taking any medications before taking magnesium.

- **Relationship to the LOVE:** Magnesium helps to keep the heart's rhythm balanced.

Potassium

This silvery-white alkaline compound is found in a wide variety of fruits and vegetables.

- **Functions:** Potassium maintains the electrical properties of cells, which connects to the function of cardiac, smooth, and skeletal muscles, as well as brain and nerve function. Supplementation may help reduce high blood pressure and the risk of stroke and cardiovascular disease.

- **Deficiency:** Deficiency can result in skin problems (severe dryness, acne), changes in gastrointestinal function (constipation, diarrhea), heart rhythm irregularities, blood pressure dysfunction, muscle weakness and fatigue, nausea, and vomiting. A number of medications can result in low potassium in the body.

- **Overuse:** Excess potassium can lead to stomach upset, nausea, weakness, low blood pressure, and heart problems.

- **Interactions:** Use of blood pressure or other medications that retain potassium in the body may lead to high levels of potassium in the body.

- **Relationship to the LOVE:** Together with other minerals like calcium and magnesium, potassium can ensure that the heart can receive and give out sufficient energy.

Blood-Lipid Support

The heart organ and web of blood vessels that extend out from it are sensitive to the amount of lipids (fats) flowing through the blood. Too much of certain types of fat, combined with the effects of high blood pressure, can lead to stress on the blood vessels, ultimately causing injury and fat infiltration into the site. Over the long term, the blood vessel wall narrows and circulation is reduced. The probability for blocked arteries and the risk for a blood clot and subsequent lack of blood flow to the heart (heart attack) increases. By keeping blood cholesterol levels low, the heart can remain active and moving. When the circulatory network is congested by fat, ask the following questions of the heart:

- What is causing blocks in my ability to love life?
- What is accumulating within my heart that no longer serves me?

Phytosterols

Phytosterols, or plant sterols (beta-sitosterol), are compounds from plants that look like cholesterol, but actually block the absorption of cholesterol in the intestine. Overall, these compounds are well tolerated, although in some individuals, they can cause nausea and gastrointestinal upset. There has been concern that phytosterols can lower absorption of fat-soluble vitamins like vitamin E and carotenoids like beta-carotene. Individuals with sitosterolemia should avoid phytosterols.

Red Yeast Rice

This nutritional product is the end result of rice fermented with *Monascus purpureus* yeast. The fermentation process produces a number of cholesterol-lowering actives, including lovastatin (a drug prescribed for cholesterol reduction). Red yeast rice supplements work in ways similar to statin drugs by inhibiting the enzyme in the body that manufactures cholesterol. If not fermented correctly, however, it can become contaminated with citrinin, a toxin that causes kidney failure. Side effects include those associated with statin drugs—liver damage, elevated liver enzymes, and muscle weakness. Red yeast rice may lower body levels of coenzyme Q10 and affect the metabolism of botanical supplements like St. John's wort. Other effects may be gastrointestinal complaints, dizziness, and allergic reactions. It may interact with several drugs. Use under the supervision of a qualified health-care professional. A dose of 2.4 g daily has been used, but cholesterol-lowering effects may occur with lower doses (1.2 g per day).

Circulation Support

The river of blood moving through your veins is important for the delivery of oxygen and nutrients to the rest of your body. Without healthy, flowing blood, stagnation can result in various parts of the body and contribute to blocks in other parts of the body. For example, if you have poor circulation to the brain, you may not get the materials you need for better thinking, memory, and concentration. Several herbs can provide important support to your circulatory system.

Bilberry Fruit Extract

The fruit and leaf of this berry (*Vaccinium myrtillus*) have a high concentration of purple pigments, anthocyanidins, that help maintain the integrity of the capillaries. It may also have blood glucose-lowering effects. Supplementation with this extract may interact with hypoglycemic supplements and drugs, ultimately requiring dosing adjustments of anti-diabetic drugs like insulin. Consult a qualified healthcare provider if you wish to supplement with bilberry and you are diabetic. See chapter 10 for more details.

Bioflavonoids

The term "bioflavonoids" refers to thousands of individual plant compounds commonly found in fruit sources, especially citrus fruits. Typical bioflavonoids in dietary supplements are quercetin and rutin. Together with vitamin C, they work to strengthen the capillaries and veins, and to promote healthy circulation of blood. Note that, if you are taking bioflavonoids from grapefruit, they may interfere with the metabolism of certain drugs. Side effects of quercetin supplementation include headache, a tingling sensation in the extremities, and kidney toxicity, while those of rutin are headache, flushing, rashes, and gastrointestinal discomfort. Quercetin is commonly recommended at 400–500 mg three times per day. A dose of 730 mg was effective in reducing blood pressure in people with high blood pressure. Rutin taken at 2 g was shown to relieve swelling due to blood vessel dysfunction.

Garlic Extract

Garlic extract is known for its ability to lower blood pressure and blood-fat levels, and reduce blood clots. Doses between 600–1200 mg daily may result in these beneficial effects. Side effects may include offensive breath and body odor, gastrointestinal discomfort, nausea, and vomiting. Exercise caution if taking other supplements or medications that have anticoagulant effects. Garlic interacts with the metabolism of a number of medications. Consult your healthcare professional before taking it. Note that odorless garlic preparations may not contain the active compound, allicin.

Gotu Kola

Gotu kola (*Centella asiatica*) has a number of effects on the body, especially for restoring blood circulation. A gotu kola extract (120–180 mg daily) has been shown to improve circulation and decrease swelling in individuals with venous insufficiency. It may cause gastrointestinal complaints, nausea, drowsiness, and liver toxicity (elevated liver enzymes). Do not use with herbs, supplements, or drugs that affect the liver or that have sedative properties.

Grapeseed Extract

Grape products, particularly grapeseed extract, are abundant in compounds that help improve chronic venous insufficiency and vein health through their antioxidant, vasodilation (blood-vessel-opening), and anti-platelet effects. Side effects include headache, gastrointestinal complaints, cough, and sore throat. There are possible interactions with supplements or drugs with anticoagulant activity, or those that lower blood pressure. An initial higher starting dose of grapeseed extract (75–300 mg) for the first couple of weeks, followed by a longer-term lower dose (40–80 mg daily) has been suggested for vein health.

Horse Chestnut

The seeds of this plant (*Aesculus hippocastanum*) are most commonly used in the treatment of chronic venous insufficiency. Side effects include dizziness, nausea, headache, itching, gastrointestinal upset, and kidney damage. Horse chestnut may cause allergic reactions in some people. It may interact with supplements or drugs with anticoagulant or hypoglycemic (blood-sugar lowering) activity. The dose for chronic venous insufficiency is a standardized extract containing 50 mg of the active, aescin, used twice daily.

Other Supplements for the LOVE

Of course, there are numerous supplements that may help your LOVE system. I'm only providing a window into some of the well-recognized ones. In this section, I review my personal favorites.

Coenzyme Q10 (CoQ10)

This fat-soluble, vitamin-like substance (*ubiquinone*) is found in all cells in the body, especially in the heart, liver, kidney, and pancreas. It functions as an antioxidant, plays a role in energy production, aids circulation of the blood, and helps stimulate immune function. CoQ10 lowers blood pressure and strengthens heart muscle. Even though the body can produce CoQ10 in small amounts, these levels are not always adequate. Statins, drugs used for cholesterol reduction, are known to reduce blood levels of coenzyme Q10. Supplementation in the range of 100–200 mg daily in two to three separate doses has been used for a variety of conditions, including heart health.

Green Food Powders

Foods like alfalfa, barley grass, broccoli powder, chlorella, chlorophyll, spirulina, and young grasses like wheat grass supply an optimal ratio of nutritious, bioavailable compounds like chlorophyll, amino acids, enzymes, and minerals like calcium, magnesium, and potassium.

Hawthorn

The leaf, fruit, and flower of hawthorn (*Crataegus laevigata*) have been used for several aspects of heart function, including reducing symptoms of heart failure and lowering cholesterol, and strengthening the heart muscle and heart rhythm. Treating people with heart failure with 900–1800 mg of a standardized extract has led to beneficial effects. Side effects include vertigo, dizziness, gastrointestinal complaints, fatigue, rash, palpitations, headache, and agitation. Hawthorn may interact with supplements and drugs that have effects on blood pressure or dilation of the blood vessels.

CHAPTER 9

THE AQUAMARINE TRUTH

One's philosophy is not best expressed in words; it is expressed in the choices one makes.

Eleanor Roosevelt

KEY WORDS FOR THE TRUTH: aquamarine, authenticity, choice, communication, coordination, expression, faith, freedom, senses, sound, speaking, surrender, truth, voice

The TRUTH system dwells deep in our throats, where much activity takes place: talking, hearing, chewing, swallowing, and breathing. The messenger of our truths—our voice—allows us to express our views, opinions, and choices. Whereas the LOVE system equips us with love and touch for healing, the TRUTH system provides us with the senses of hearing, smell, and taste. With these senses, our life experiences are made real and we can learn and make choices to direct our paths.

The TRUTH system also provides us a place where we can be vulnerably powerful. We make ourselves known through our personal truths. At your core, who are you and what do you stand for? What does your true self look like? The TRUTH system welcomes you to use the courage of the heart to express your beliefs, opinions, feelings, and thoughts. It gives you the tool of will to move in the direction of your authenticity.

The TRUTH and Your Body

The TRUTH system represents the throat and the anatomy surrounding the throat, including the larynx, pharynx, thyroid, neck, upper esophagus, chin, tongue, lips, mouth, ears, and nose. The ability of the nose to smell, the tongue to taste, and the ears to hear are all contained within the TRUTH system, which makes it essential for our connection to food. We experience food by smelling and tasting it, chewing it and coating it with saliva—which assists in the breakdown of certain nutrients—and finally, by swallowing it and making it accessible to the rest of the body. The TRUTH system is a gateway for taking in food. It also governs, to a great extent, how we process our food, since it contains the thyroid, the gland responsible for how we metabolize what we take in.

The Truth and Eating

The TRUTH system ties in intimately to our authentic connection with food and equips us with the tools we need to process it—chewing, tasting, hearing, and speaking. It enriches our relationship with food and eating. It comprises a dense area of our physiology, with much activity happening all at once. It is important that we make the best food and eating choices to support this system.

Here are some questions to help you determine if you are maximizing the function of your TRUTH system.

Are you tapping into your senses with foods?
We are sensory beings. We take in sensory information and process it on many levels. For the FLOW system, we depend on sensory input for pleasure. For the FIRE system, we receive messages from our environment to integrate within our own energy and body. The LOVE system takes in a huge amount of emotional information even before an interaction has taken place. The TRUTH system represents a practical manifestation of the sensory tools we have, and all of those sensors are engaged when we eat.

Your ears give you the capacity to listen intently to communication about eating, whether listening for animals to hunt in the wild or responding to the screeching of the tea kettle on the stove. What do you hear as you shop at the grocery store? Some use sound to help with food selection: for example, shaking melons or pounding gently on an acorn squash. In the more subtle background, your sensory experience of eating may be colored by hearing statements in your unconscious mind when you make food choices: "I *should* really have the salmon and not the rib-eye steak." Or "My mom would want me to eat *right.*" Or "What would Jack say if he knew I indulged in rocky road ice cream?"

Sometimes, you can almost hear a person's message resonating in your ears. The TRUTH system encourages you to listen to your own voice when it comes to food and eating—what is real for *you*—rather than taking on external messages from others.

What about the communication that occurs in the course of eating a meal that indicates we are enjoying eating? Sometimes, we resort to making sounds while eating to convey our enjoyment. Think of the soup ad that proclaims: "Mmmmgood!" Or the strong slurping noise that is common in Japanese culture to voice approval for a tasty soup. Somehow, the sounds we make add to our experience of eating. While eating in a group, we also hear comments about how flavorful the food is: "Isn't this cake the best you've ever tasted?" Or "I've never had a peach so juicy!" Our auditory input certainly adds to our experience of eating. Kendra comments that she gets the most satisfaction from positive feedback about the pumpkin pie she makes every Thanksgiving. These words nourish her in much the same way that her pumpkin pie gives delight to her family members.

The dynamic interface of the nose, lips, mouth, and tongue furnishes us with a network of sensory receptors that all work together to give us immediate feedback. Once you smell food, salivation begins and digestive juices start to squirt into your stomach. Your nose and tongue work in tandem. Without smell, we lose our ability to taste food. George was born without the ability to smell, so he was unable to taste food. For him, eating became much more about the textures of food. He liked steak because of the chewy texture and the feeling of fullness he had after eating it. Perhaps you have experienced this sensation temporarily when you had a cold. Think of how having a stuffy nose made eating less enjoyable and how tasty foods became when you felt better!

Do you chew food thoroughly and well?

I have heard many a parent in a restaurant gently reprimanding their children to slow down and chew their food. When we are busy, it is easy to slip into the mode of gulping our food down to save time. Some even like to drink their food, consuming high-protein shakes. However, we experience different physiological responses when chewing, as opposed to simply swallowing, food. When we chew food, we unlock its messages gradually. We enter into a greater, more complex relationship with the food in its natural state. On the other hand, when we drink food like a fruit smoothie, we get different messages. The signals from the food are quickly assimilated into our physiology, and the matrix of the food is altered. This change isn't necessarily detrimental; it is simply a different translation of what the food has in store for us.

How you eat says volumes about your TRUTH system. When you eat quickly, without chewing with consciousness, you deny yourself the richness of the eating experience. Chances are that eating quickly will only make you hungry later, as you are not gathering the full authenticity of the eating experience. Also, you may develop indigestion followed by fatigue because you are burdening your lower digestive tract. Breaking food apart into smaller bits helps your FIRE system transform these bits into powerful energy. Indeed, the mouth is where the digestive process starts and where much of the starch digestion occurs. You can help all your systems of health when you begin the eating process by chewing thoroughly.

Do you integrate your TRUTH system activities?

Since the TRUTH system is packed with all types of activities, it helps to ensure that they are synchronized in a way that is balanced. When you take in big gulps of food and swallow while breathing erratically, you develop hiccups. You have likely heard the phrase: "Don't talk with your mouth full." If you are busy talking and listening, you may not be able to focus on tasting or chewing your food thoroughly. When eating, establish a rhythm. No chewing or swallowing while talking. And connect your breath to the bites of food you take.

Once you place your awareness in the proper coordination of activities while you eat, your TRUTH system will fall into balance and your food will enter the transformative process properly.

Do you eat with authenticity and respect?

The LOVE system is largely about gratitude and—as it relates to food and eating—giving thanks for a meal. The TRUTH system literally voices this gratitude through spoken words, prayers, and intentions. The reverence and dignity we have for nature and the provision of foods manifests into other areas of our lives. Some traditions honor respectful eating practices by consuming foods blessed by a spiritual person, or by only eating certain foods on designated days.

Do you eat in harmony with your metabolism?

We all have our own rhythm. Some people tell me straight out that they are not morning people and breakfast is not appetizing at all. Others comment that they have a certain time of the day when they usually get hungry. It is meaningful to honor your own body's circadian rhythm and your own eating patterns. You have to discern, however, whether you have these patterns because you habitually eat in a certain way—repeatedly eating high-glycemic-index sugary foods that drain your energy, causing you to crave more every couple of hours—or whether your body has these patterns hard-wired into it. There are a number of studies on the benefits of breakfast. If you have difficulty eating breakfast, perhaps there are some ways to compromise—for instance, having a small piece of fruit rather than a large vegetable-and-egg scramble.

Try to step back and observe your body's eating rhythm. Shift your schedule on certain days to see whether the pattern is inherent in you or merely a function of your lifestyle. By doing so, you honor the rhythm and balance of your thyroid gland, one of the master regulators of your metabolism.

Are you making high-quality eating choices?

Fortunately, we have choice. Moreover, our small and big choices cause a ripple effect in our lives, the lives of others, and the state of the planet. The act of eating is an important choice we make every day. As I mentioned previously, an average person makes close to 84,000 decisions about food in a lifetime. How many of those decisions make you feel good? When you are confronted with food choices, what factors go into making your choice? Cost? Convenience? Taste? Health? Maybe it varies depending on the moment.

Your TRUTH system is largely about making the best choice in every moment. It is about a good, quality decision that is well thought-out or well felt. If you have the opportunity to eat organically, do you? Should you? Are you concerned about genetically modified organisms (GMOs)? You may want to explore these questions for yourself to see where you resonate. There are several layers of high-quality eating. For instance, if health is your guiding light when it comes to food purchases, and if you have a craving for chocolate, think about a high-quality bar with high cocoa percentage rather than the milk chocolate bar loaded with grams of sugar and dairy. In this way, you honor your body's need while presenting it with the healthiest option available. In essence: You *can* have your cake and eat it too!

Do you aim for variety?

The TRUTH system is experiential and uses the senses of hearing, taste, and smell to maximize its experience in the external world. It's important to get a variety of foods in your diet. As we saw in the ROOT chapter, most people settle into what I refer to as "eating ruts," or established eating patterns that can provide a numbing experience. When you eat the same food(s) all the time, you also have a greater chance of developing a food sensitivity or allergy. This is your body's protective mechanism encouraging stability through variety.

What brings your TRUTH system to life is an assortment of colors, tastes, and smells to soothe it. Presenting yourself with a palette of options provides you with the ability to both choose and experience. The Ayurvedic approach to eating, which encourages a balance of hot and cold foods mixed with spicy, sour, sweet, bitter, and astringent flavors, is a perfect way to balance a meal.

On the other hand, variety needs to be kept in check. Too much variety may lead to binge eating. Luxurious buffets are known for prompting excessive eating. Provocative research has shown that the same amount of food spread into several small bowls at a party versus one or two large bowls results in more snacking by party-goers. Other consumer research by Kahn and Wansink found that just three more colors of M&Ms in a bowl can lead to more munching (an average of forty-three more M&Ms).

Overall, the "right" amount of variety keeps you satisfied and prevents you from overeating (too much variety) and from developing food sensitivities and allergies (too little variety).

Eating Activities for the TRUTH

1. Try the simple practice of chewing your food carefully and slowly until it becomes liquid in your mouth. Focus on creating an abundance of saliva in your mouth, thinking of it as liquid transformative juice. With each bite, see what messages the food is giving you. What insight do you receive? You can also make this an active exercise by infusing messages into every bite of food.

2. Allow yourself to listen to the messages of food. Pick a food that you feel drawn to and create a journal dialogue with it.

3. Visit an ethnic grocery store and pick one new food to try.

4. Where do you lack respect for yourself and become inauthentic in your eating habits? Create a statement of authenticity that is simple to remember. For example: I feed my body the best I can in the moment.

5. The next time you are eating with others, observe the balance you have between talking, chewing, and breathing. Are they synchronized? If not, focus on anchoring yourself in your breath and chew in the breathing rhythm.

6. Pay attention to the importance of your sense of smell when eating. Does smell add to your experience of eating?

7. Note language used around food. How do you express your hunger with words? Your feelings of satisfaction with eating? What words are used on the packaging of what you eat? Are those messages you choose for your life?

Foods for Your TRUTH

In Appendix A, I assign a symbol to each of the seven systems of health. The symbol I chose for the TRUTH system is a five-pointed star. Aside from the fact that it is the fifth system of health, it also represents the complexity of the five senses: smell, hearing, taste, sight, and touch. Finally, the five points also speak to the five tastes of food that we are capable of distinguishing with our tongues: salty, sweet, bitter, sour, and savory (umami). I like to think of foods that are moistening and provide a diverse palette of tastes as those that are good for the TRUTH system.

Sea Plants

Plants derived from the sea—like nori, agar, dulse, hijiki, arame, and kelp—are excellent sources of nourishment for the thyroid gland. Many people in Western society aren't familiar with edible sea plants other than the pressed sheet of nori in which sushi is rolled. However, in other countries, particularly Japan, sea plants are a staple of the diet. These magnificent plants are rich in minerals from the sea—including iodine, which is a nutrient that plays a role in proper functioning of the thyroid gland, helping to regulate our metabolism. Goiter, or an enlargement of the thyroid gland in the throat, develops when you do not have enough iodine in your diet.

Soups

Soups represent the fusion between an earth-based food and the element of water. Both hot and cold soups are wholesome combinations to support the TRUTH system. The nice thing about soups is that they take time to eat. Usually, you eat them one spoonful or sip at a time, creating more mindfulness and integration in your eating experience.

One way I like to bring together the LOVE and TRUTH systems is through what I call "gratitude bites." Before you bring in a forkful or spoonful of food, say to yourself: "thank you." This gesture of gratitude keeps you in the moment, slows down your eating, and fills your heart as you eat. Try it, even if it's just for a few bites!

Sauces, Dressings, and Marinades

I am not typically a fan of store-bought sauces and dressings, because they are typically laden with chemicals, dyes, and sweeteners. However, there are wonderfully nourishing and tasty sauces you can make to add some cohesion and moisture to your meals. For example, mix tahini (sesame seed butter) with a little oil (sesame oil or extra-virgin olive oil) and perhaps some lemon juice and herbs to drizzle over vegetables or a grilled chicken breast. Or perhaps you like organic tamari sauce on vegetables and/or meats. The goal of a sauce is not to be excessive, but rather to unify and integrate the components of a dish. Just a small amount may make salmon more moist and palatable, or grilled vegetables more satisfying. Marinades, especially those incorporating apple cider vinegar, lime juice, and lemon juice are perfect for making meats tender, as they begin the breakdown process before it even hits your mouth!

Juices

Much like store-bought sauces, dressings, and marinades, juices can also be unhealthy, since they capture just the sugar part of the fruit rather than the whole food. I believe the value of juices depends on how they are used. They can be consumed excessively, bringing in high amounts of sugar. However, they can also provide a great way to get colorful phytonutrients and to moisten the throat. I think juices should be sipped during a meal in smaller quantities, around two to four fluid ounces—enough so that food mixes well in your mouth and goes down nicely. There are some interesting studies on beet juice, pomegranate juice, and other types of whole-food-based juices that have health benefits.

SMOOTHIES

I'm all for smoothies! Even my "junk food" dad loves a green smoothie in the morning. The beauty of smoothies is that they are like a meal: nutrient-dense and high in calories. And they can provide a complex mixture of fiber, carbohydrate, healthy fat (like coconut oil or almond milk), and even quality protein (like rice, pea, or organic soy-based protein). The downside of smoothies is that they can be too "quick" as a meal. We guzzle them down, but we may not feel full. It's best to "chew" your smoothie, treating it as food. Make sure you go slowly, take your time, and let your mouth—the starting place of the TRUTH system—do its initial digestive work.

Ethnic Foods

As a fun exercise, I like to have clients experiment with ethnic foods of their own heritage and explore the origin of those foods and meals. This activity forces them to talk to their tribe about the history of their meals. At first mention of this task, Carol was a bit apprehensive, as she was choosing to eat raw foods and thought that most ethnic foods involved cooking. However, when she took the time to go to some Asian grocery stores, she found some delightful foods like lychees. She enjoyed the perfume-like taste of the lychee flesh and decided to incorporate it into her food selection.

Eating ethnic foods allows you to bring a stream of variety into your habitual world, and to experience the truth of eating within other cultures. When you eat these foods, you connect with the people and the culture where they are eaten and grown. You tap into a huge reservoir of knowledge and experience that you might not otherwise have known.

Fruits

High-water fruits like watermelon, cucumber, cantaloupe, and grapes can serve the TRUTH system by providing sufficient moisture to open the throat to make it easier to speak the truth. Astringent or sour fruits like lemon, lime, and kiwi pucker and activate the throat as well.

Supplements for Your TRUTH

The TRUTH system governs choice. And that freedom of choice extends to your decision of whether or not to take supplements. Do you actively choose to take certain supplements or do you allow others—the media, vendors, other individuals—to make that selection for you? To decide whether taking supplemental forms of nutrients is beneficial for your physiology, tune into your body's wisdom for your ultimate answer. Work with a healthcare professional for clarity and focus.

And remember to bring your full awareness as you take supplements. Swallowing a pill or chugging down a spoonful of liquid is easy for some individuals and, as a result, taking supplements may become automatic or routine. I believe that it's essential to be fully present when taking supplements.

Forms and Variety of Supplements

Supplements and botanicals come in a variety of forms, including tablets, capsules, liquid, softgels, chewables, and powders. It may not always be practical (or easy) to swallow large tablets. Sometimes certain nutrients are more bioavailable in liquid form. Likewise, eating a chewable may allow the nutrient to be absorbed within the mouth cavity. Allow your TRUTH system the flexibility of choice and refrain from becoming stagnant with any single delivery system.

Taking in the same supplements every day can cause your body to become programmed. It may be worthwhile to consider changing your supplement routine regularly, so that your body does not become too attached to any particular dietary supplement. Getting the right dose for a defined period of time may help your body respond to it more effectively. Work with your healthcare professional to alternate or rotate your supplements.

Vitamins and Minerals

If you are feeling that you need just a bit more support for your TRUTH beyond what soups, stews, sauces, fruit juices, teas, and moist fruits can do for you, you may want to explore integrating some of the vitamins and minerals listed below into your eating routine.

Vitamin A

Vitamin A (retinol) deficiency can occur together with iodine deficiency, leading to impaired thyroid function. In studies with children who are iodine- and vitamin A-deficient, vitamin A supplementation helps the body to use iodine from iodized salt. See chapter 5 for more details. Selenium may also have a role to play here and you can read more on page 162.

Vitamin D

The four parathyroid glands are nestled next to the thyroid gland, yet they do not have the same function as the thyroid gland. Their job is to ensure that there is an adequate level of calcium in the body. To accomplish this task, they release parathyroid hormone to help activate vitamin D in the body so it can stimulate calcium absorption in the gut. The parathyroid glands start making more of their hormone if vitamin D levels are too low, causing a condition called hyperparathyroidism. If you are deficient in vitamin D (your practitioner can do a lab test), it may be worthwhile to consider supplementation. See chapter 5 for more details.

Iodine

Iodine is an essential nutrient in foods grown in soil or harvested from the sea, or in foods with added iodine like iodized salt.

- **Functions:** Iodine concentrates in the thyroid gland and is used to make iodine-rich hormones that control many physiological processes, like metabolism.
- **Deficiency:** Iodine deficiency has serious effects on brain development and is associated with mental retardation. The classic deficiency symptom is goiter, or enlarged thyroid gland.
- **Overuse:** Too much iodine results in a burning sensation in the mouth and throat, sore teeth and gums, a metallic taste in the mouth, and gastric upset.
- **Interactions:** Discuss iodine supplementation with a healthcare practitioner if you are taking thyroid medications.
- **Relationship to the TRUTH:** With too little iodine, the thyroid gland can become sluggish. On the other hand, there may be some thyroid gland conditions where iodine is not indicated. Check with your healthcare professional.

Selenium

The thyroid gland has the highest concentration of selenium in the body, as it is needed for the manufacture and metabolism of thyroid hormones. Specifically, it is a cofactor for the enzyme that converts one thyroid hormone (T4, thyroxine) into another (T3, triiodothyronine), a reaction that does not happen efficiently in hypothyroidism. In the case of iodine deficiency, selenium deficiency can worsen hypothyroidism. While there is still active discussion on this topic, one study indicated that taking 200 mcg selenium daily helped to reduce blood levels of a marker of autoimmune thyroiditis (called anti-thyroid peroxidase). See chapter 6 for more details.

Thyroid Gland and Throat Support

The thyroid gland, nestled in the TRUTH vicinity, is one of the main focal points for the control of metabolism throughout the body. Whereas the FIRE system contains the organs of transformation and energy exchange, the TRUTH system provides the framework and coordinates the secretion of hormones for those processes to occur. It also determines how the entire body (not just the digestive organs) integrate the energy harvested.

The throat is a vessel for expression. It allows for breath to be inhaled and exhaled, for food to be swallowed and accepted, and for the voice to form and exit. When troubled with expressing certain thoughts, feelings, or opinions, your throat may become dry, which may even develop into a sore throat or tonsilitis, especially if you are inflamed about something. It is important to keep the throat moist and lubricated for the flow of expression.

Below are several supplements that support the thyroid gland and throat, helping to balance your TRUTH system.

Licorice

Licorice (*Glycyrrhiza glabra*) has a number of properties that make it desirable to take for a sore throat. In addition to its ability to help clear mucus, it can also soothe and coat the throat. For a sore throat, it can be prepared as a tea by steeping 1 tsp. of licorice root in hot water for two to three minutes. or by sucking on a slice of raw licorice. Do not use licorice in pregnancy. Excess amounts over an extended period (several weeks) can lead to changes in sodium and fluid levels, electrolyte imbalance, and elevations in blood pressure. Avoid using licorice with antihypertensives, anticoagulants, corticosteroids, and estrogens. It may have estrogenic effects, so do not take if a hormone-sensitive condition is present.

Marshmallow

The root and leaf of the marshmallow plant (*Althaea officinalis*) have been used as a traditional remedy for sore throat. It contains mucilages to coat the throat and help suppress cough. It is typically prepared as a tea using either the dried leaf or dried root. It should not be taken by pregnant or lactating women. It may reduce blood sugar and lead to increased urination (diuretic). Use caution when taking with supplements or drugs that have blood-sugar-lowering action or those that may be affected by increased excretion in urine. Take marshmallow root or leaf separate from other medications, as it is known to impair drug absorption in the gut.

Sea Kelp/Bladderwrack

Sea plants like brown seaweed (*Fucus vesiculosus*) are nourishing for the TRUTH system due to their iodine content. Note that sea plants are also prone to concentrating heavy metals found in the sea, like cadmium and arsenic. Too much can lead to hypo- or hyper-thyroidism (similar to the effects of iodine). Consult with a healthcare practitioner before taking with medications for the thyroid gland or anticoagulant drugs.

Slippery Elm

The inner bark rind from this North American deciduous tree (*Ulmus rubra*) contains mucilages (or long chains of sugars complexed with protein) that, when taken orally, provide a soothing film over mucous membranes like the throat. Slippery elm is often taken in the form of lozenges and used for sore throats and coughs. Pregnant and lactating women should avoid it.

Soy

Even though soy protein helps prevent cardiovascular disease (see chapter 8), it may reduce the production of thyroid hormone in individuals who have thyroid problems, and especially in those who have iodine deficiency (see Iodine on page 162). For those with iodine deficiency and thyroid issues, limit the consumption of soy.

Allergy and Sinus Support

Conditions like allergies involve both the ROOT (immune) and TRUTH (sinus) systems. Allergic rhinitis (often called nasal allergies or hay fever) is a specific expression of the allergy category. When the immune system becomes over-reactive to environmental substances like animal dander, dust, mold, or plant pollen, the TRUTH system is affected with an array of symptoms, including coughing, headache, itchy nose, throat, or mouth, irritated skin and eyes, runny nose, inability to smell, sneezing, sore throat, and wheezing. Allergic sinusitis calls us to examine what we are overreacting to in our environment.

Blue-Green Algae

Blue-green algae (*Spirulina platensis*) is a complex mixture of single-celled organisms from the sea. It contains a variety of nutrients, including protein, B vitamins, fat, and minerals. It has been shown to stimulate immune function and reduce symptoms of allergic reactions. Taking a specific spirulina supplement at 2 g daily for twelve weeks led to a reduction of an inflammatory marker (interleukin-4) in individuals with allergic rhinitis. Ensure that the supplement is free of toxic blue-green species contaminants. These contaminants can produce toxic liver substances that can result in death. Do not take if you have an autoimmune disease or take immunosuppressants. Side effects include gastrointestinal complaints.

Butterbur

The leaf, rhizome, and root of butterbur (*Petasites hybridus*) may be useful in reducing symptoms of allergic rhinitis. Supplementation with specific butterbur extracts that do not contain toxic compounds that naturally occur in the plant (pyrrolizidine alkaloids) have been shown to be effective for improving nasal symptoms. It appears to lower compounds related to the immune response (e.g., histamines, leukotrienes) in the blood of individuals with allergic rhinitis. Specific butterbur extracts are available for short-term use for relief of allergic rhinitis symptoms. It may also be effective for migraines. Side effects include belching, headaches, itchy eyes, diarrhea, asthma, and fatigue. Some individuals may be allergic to this plant family. Taking butterbur may influence the metabolism of certain drugs. Confirm that the extract is free of alkaloids.

Common Cold

Whereas allergies are due to a hyperactive immune system, the common cold can result when immune defenses are low in the presence of a viral invader. Supplements discussed in chapter 5 for supporting immune function—particularly vitamin C, zinc, and echinacea—can assist the TRUTH system in combating cold symptoms.

Quercetin and Bromelain

Quercetin supplementation at 250–600 mg three times daily, taken five to ten minutes before meals, may be helpful for calming the inflammatory-immune response with allergies. It has been suggested that quercetin may work more effectively if taken together with the pineapple enzyme bromelain (400–500 mg three times daily of an 1800–2000 mcu potency bromelain). Side effects of bromelain include allergic reactions in those with pineapple allergy and gastrointestinal disturbances. Use caution if taking together with other supplements or drugs that have anticoagulant effects. Zinc may inhibit the activity of bromelain, so take them separately. See chapter 6 for more details.

Stinging Nettle

The above-ground parts of the stinging nettle plant (*Urtica dioica*) have traditionally been used for allergies and allergic rhinitis. It appears to work best when taken at the start of symptoms, and may be beneficial because of its quercetin content. Quercetin has anti-inflammatory effects and dampens the release of histamine from immune cells. Side effects include gastrointestinal complaints, sweating, and allergic skin reactions. Nettle may interact with the activity of supplements or drugs taken concurrently that have effects on blood pressure, blood sugar, central nervous system (CNS) depression, fluid excretion, and coagulation. The typical dose for allergic rhinitis is 300 mg three times daily.

Jaw Support

Temporomandibular joint (TMJ) problems indicate tightness and constriction in the jaw muscles. TMJ issues may evolve into an inflammatory condition like osteoarthritis. With TMJ osteoarthritis, nutritional supplementation for joint support may be helpful. If you have TMJ issues, ask yourself: What am I not saying? Instead of vocalizing your thoughts, you may feel more comfortable expressing them in some other way, like journaling, singing, or developing a personal mantra that can support you.

Glucosamine Sulfate

In a study with people with TMJ osteoarthritis, glucosamine sulfate at 500 mg taken three times daily was found to be more effective at reducing pain compared with those taking ibuprofen.

Sensory Support

The TRUTH system provides you with a gateway to the external world through the senses of hearing, smelling, and tasting. If any of these senses are not functioning properly, examine whether there is a block or barrier preventing you from taking in your surroundings or experiencing and interacting with life. Two key minerals are most useful for supporting these senses—magnesium and zinc.

Magnesium

As demonstrated in human and animal studies, magnesium supplementation, even at low doses, may prevent noise-induced hearing loss. See chapter 8 for more details.

Zinc

Zinc supplementation (25–100 mg) may help with taste dysfunction (a condition called hypogeusia) in people who have low zinc levels. It may also improve taste in those with various taste disorders due to medications, radiation, and post-trauma. See chapter 5 for more details.

CHAPTER 10

THE INDIGO INSIGHT

Be curious always, for knowledge will not acquire you; you must acquire it.

Sudie Back

KEY WORDS FOR THE INSIGHT: concentration, dreams, illusion, imagination, indigo, insight, intuition, mood, perception, sleep, spiral, thought, vision, visualization, wisdom

With the INSIGHT system, we begin to separate truth from illusion. Simply put, with our inner "sight," we can glean from our panoramic experience of life what we need to learn and how we need to grow. When you are fully opened to your INSIGHT, you have the tools of awareness needed to expose you to a deep knowing of who you truly are and what your path of life entails. A healthy INSIGHT system will be consistent with following your internal visions and dreams. When life is aligned with your inner knowing, your thoughts and actions are resolute.

We engage our INSIGHT systems whenever our minds are involved—when we engage in heavy thought and reverie, sleep deeply, or dream. Dreams are important messengers, as they usually embody symbolic, valuable, and meaningful truths that we can apply to waking life. Because of the infinite power that we receive through our inner intuition, we can easily become overwhelmed. However, when we are able to watch our thoughts like clouds, allowing them to flow through us rather than sticking to us like cotton candy, we feel healthier and more free. We release ourselves from being prisoners of our minds and in our everyday lives, and begin to separate fact from fiction. It is helpful to view life as a movie, watching it unfold in front of you, rather than becoming stuck on or attached to a certain part of it. This is the true wisdom of your INSIGHT system.

The INSIGHT and Your Body

The INSIGHT system includes the eyes, the forehead, and the pituitary gland, which controls the clockwork of our endocrine gland secretions. It is the center that balances and integrates hormones in the body. The INSIGHT oversees the brain and thoughts, and therefore is directly linked to the production and workings of neurotransmitters like serotonin and dopamine. Through this connection, the INSIGHT system is largely responsible for our moods and for the projected personality of the self.

The INSIGHT and Eating

One of the features I find missing in peoples' daily eating is their intuition. We tend to become too focused and fixated on the intellectual aspects of eating, which often come from the outside, rather than the inside. Here are some questions to ask yourself about the relationship between your INSIGHT and how you eat.

Do you eat intuitively?

In chapter 5, we discussed questioning the body about its food needs, an active process designed to help you better read and dialogue with your physiology. Intuitive eating can be both an active and a passive process. Sometimes you may feel strongly at the gut level that you need to eat certain foods. Perhaps you suddenly have a strong feeling that your body would do well with having some steamed spinach. During and after eating the spinach, you experience a sense of alignment within your being. You may feel more resonant and more vibrant.

At other times, you may simply intuit what you need to eat. Maybe you are looking over a restaurant menu with a variety of choices, wondering what to order. You can certainly ask your body what it needs and begin that conscious conversation. Alternately, you can focus within and ask to be guided to the dish on the menu that may be in congruence with your health. You may be surprised by what you are led to eat! It is important to learn how to listen to, trust, and honor your eating intuition. The more you listen, the more readily it will speak to you!

When you are not in sync with your intuition, you may find yourself facing "analysis-paralysis" when it comes to eating. Over-intellectualizing eating by reducing it to calories or grams of macronutrients, or crafting eating habits based on trends, squelches your intuitive wisdom. Rather than have your intuition be boxed in by the structure of what and how you are eating, embrace the deep resounding intuition spiraling from within your subconscious.

Do you have food addictions?

Some individuals may feel that they are addicted to eating certain foods. This addiction surpasses the occasional craving and takes a strong hold on their being. It becomes the commander of their INSIGHT system. One common food addiction is sugary foods, as they provide an energy surge to send our neuron synapses firing in all directions. Maybe there is a specific food item that you do not feel you can mentally escape—chocolate is a popular one.

One way to gain insight into a food addiction is to look inside. When you understand your deeper connection to the food, you can more easily overcome the addiction. Have someone you trust say the name of the food to which you are addicted over and over, usually about twenty times. Every time you hear the word, say the first word that comes to your mind; have the other person write it down. Proceed very quickly, without judgment. At the end of the exercise, look for a pattern or create a story from the twenty words. Keep your eyes closed when doing this exercise so that you can focus within and be free of any external distraction. The person guiding you should only be writing down your responses and not commenting on them. If you find that your mind is blank and nothing comes forth, sit until a word, feeling, or thought arises. When you give yourself time by being patient, your intuition often reveals the answer.

When I engage a group of clients in a workshop setting, I often ask for a volunteer with a strong food addiction and, together, we unravel the rationale behind it. I have witnessed several fascinating discoveries around food addictions, from childhood memories to a call for something greater in someone's life. For example, one person's intense attraction to ice cream was connected to her innate loneliness. When she was a child, she often went with children in the neighborhood in the summertime to the local ice cream shop. As an adult, she felt isolated and was subconsciously eating ice cream as a way to resurrect the memory of community and friendship. She had no idea of this relationship between the two until she did this activity.

Do you nourish your brain and mood?

A distinct relationship exists between food and mood: our foods can influence our moods, and our moods can certainly drive our food choices. You have most likely heard of the connection between sugar and hyperactivity in children. The brain uses glucose as a source of fuel. When it is inundated with sugar, it has lots of energy to put out.

Conversely, eating turkey or drinking warm milk may cause you to feel sleepy. As you remember from chapter 5, these foods are highly grounding. They slow your body's reactions and stabilize you. Moreover, they cause your brain chemistry to change. For example, turkey contains the amino acid tryptophan, which is the building block for serotonin, the neurotransmitter in the brain that gives us that "feel good" sensation.

Your moods may also compel you to eat in a certain way. As we discussed in chapter 6, if you do not feel your emotions, you may end up burying them into food and eating. Whereas emotions are raw and short-lived, moods slip over us like a sheath. Your moods may dictate that you eat chocolate for days on end. Or maybe you "are in the mood" for lemon sorbet three meals in a row.

The INSIGHT system is intimately connected to both the LOVE and the FLOW systems. The fats and oils discussed in chapter 6 are major constituents of brain matter. Your thoughts and behavior are strongly governed by the amount of essential fat in your brain. When you do not have enough emotional flow coming through, your LOVE and INSIGHT systems suffer. For the INSIGHT, this state manifests as depression. Eating healthy fat can encourage more fluidity in the body, from the FLOW system up to the INSIGHT system, helping to release you from depression.

Are you eating to enhance concentration?

Concentration, which falls under the auspices of the INSIGHT system, can be improved significantly by eating. When you have to study for a test or complete a physical task, your brain is active. Food provides the energy that you need to feed the brain so that you can maintain your focus. Refraining from eating foods or beverages that stimulate the brain may be beneficial for people who have difficulty concentrating.

Do you eat to improve your sleep patterns?

When you overtax your mind, you may use food to unwind it, particularly after a long day at work. Many people who engage in uncontrollable nighttime snacking can throw off the balance of their INSIGHT systems, including their sleep patterns, circadian rhythms, and delicate hormone cycles. The quality and quantity of your sleep can be improved by shifting your eating cycles into a rhythm that works for you. Most people sleep soundly when they do not eat for two or three hours before bed. If you eat right before you go to sleep, your brain (and gut) may remain too active, keeping you unsettled throughout the night. On the other hand, having a light protein snack right before bedtime may help give you a deeper, grounded quality of sleep.

You may also find that eating closer to bedtime or eating certain foods in the evening impacts the quality and intensity of your dreams. Eating foods high in sugar or caffeine in the evening puts the brain into overdrive during the sleeping hours, creating vivid dreams—and in some, even nightmares. For restful dreams, curtail nighttime eating.

Eating Activities for the INSIGHT

1. Before you start eating, clear your mind by meditating for five minutes. Empty all the thoughts you don't want to affect your eating.

2. Create a haiku or mantra that you can use to focus and harness your mental energy around your relationship with foods. For example, if you obsess about the quantity of food you eat and find yourself within a web of condemning thoughts after a meal, push your INSIGHT reset button with a mantra such as: "I eat as much as I need."

3. Practice using your intuition to make food choices when you are at the market. What do you hear? What do you see? Are these sensory signals triggers to direct your attention?

4. Do an experiment investigating the relationship between foods and your dreams. Note whether you dream about any particular foods. What significance does that food have for you? How do the foods you eat change your dreams?

5. Are you a victim of analysis-paralysis when it comes to foods? Do you allow your life to be run by "nutrition-by-number"—counting up calories, grams of fat, etc.? Try journaling to dialogue with the inner nutritional accountant that may live within your mind.

6. How is your mood affected by foods? Do you feel happy when you eat certain foods? Fatigued and depressed when you eat others? Keep a brief log of how foods affect your mood before and after you eat them.

7. How can you zoom out of your individual eating experience and connect to the expanse of the greater planetary consciousness of eating? What activities can you do to assist others in being fed (e.g., participate in a soup kitchen) or to support the sanctity of the food supply (e.g., donate to organizations that advocate organic farming practices)? Brainstorm ideas to help grow the healthy global consciousness of eating and act on one every season of the year.

8. Do you have an addiction to any particular food? What is the root of the addiction? A memory? A feeling? A thought?

Foods for Your INSIGHT

Foods for the INSIGHT system are usually more intense, concentrated foods that create a dramatic physiological and/or psychological response when only a small amount is consumed. Of course, with the INSIGHT system and its potential toward a thought-obsessive nature, the response of these foods in the body may be so overwhelming that they may become rather dizzying and addictive (going round and round). At other times, they may be more mentally insightful, protective, and stimulating. The wisdom of the INSIGHT system allows us to choose foods that can be used for either their mentally calming or their stimulating qualities.

Flavonoids

Benzodiazepines like diazepam (Valium) are well-known drugs that help people feel calmer through their sedating, hypnotic, anti-anxiety, and muscle-relaxant effects. These effects are thought to occur in part because of the drug's ability to enhance the neurotransmitter gamma-aminobutyric acid (GABA) at a specific receptor site in the brain. Certain members of the class of phytochemicals in foods, called flavonoids, seem to work through a mechanism similar to that of benzodiazepines: they are able to pass the "picky" blood-brain barrier and sit on brain receptors.

One of the first research studies published on plant flavonoids binding to these anti-anxiety receptors came from a Danish group back in 1988. They were able to identify one of the most active compounds in Karmel-itergeist, an alcoholic extract of lemon balm, nutmeg, cinnamon, and angelica root. This flavonoid was called amentoflavon(e), and it was as potent as diazepam (Valium) in binding to certain brain receptors. Since then, the large family of flavonoids has been explored and some popular types have been identified, including kaempferol, myricetin, quercetin, apigenin, luteolin, hesperetin, naringenin, catechins, epicatechins, antho-cyanidins, and cyanidins. Select flavonoids from botanicals have been reported to influence brain receptors, including:

- Apigenin, from an extract of dried flowers of *Matricaria chamomilla L.*
- Apigenin, from the dried flower heads of *Matricaria recutita L.* (asteraceae)
- Baicalein from *Scutellaria baicalensis*
- Chrysin, from the traditional medicine plant *Passiflora coerulea L.*
- Epigallocatechin gallate, which is concentrated in green tea
- Flavones from an extract of sage leaves (*Salvia officinalis L.*)
- Flavonoid glycosides in ginkgo biloba extract
- Gabrol from licorice (*Glycyrrhiza glabra*)

- Quercetin and kaempferol in linden flowers
- Quercetin in heather

Anti-anxiety drugs like benzodiazepines have many side effects, including sedation, amnesia, and ataxia, which is why some researchers are exploring safer options. In fact, one animal study suggested that, in contrast to diazepam, flavonoids like chrysin and apigenin have no amnesia-like effect on learning tasks even at higher doses than needed. In fact, apigenin had a slight enhancing effect on training-session performance.

Overall, cell and animal research has shown that flavonoids found in foods and herbs may have beneficial effects for brain and nerve health. We still don't know whether these results translate to humans, but until we know the definitive answer, it may be worthwhile to add more flavonoid-containing foods to your everyday diet.

FOODS AND MOODS

Here are some examples of the foods found to be highest in flavonoids, listed in descending order of dosage (mg of flavonoids per 100 g of the fresh weight of the edible portion) by the USDA. For more details on the flavonoid content of foods, consult the USDA Nutrient Database at *ars. usda.gov*.

- Cacao beans: 8606 mg
- Elderberries, juice concentrate: 520 mg
- Elderberries, raw: 518 mg
- Blackberry, juice concentrate: 355 mg
- Raspberries, black, raw: 324 mg
- Bilberries, raw: 289 mg
- Cocoa, dry, unsweetened: 261 mg
- Carob flour: 236 mg
- Parsley, fresh: 233 mg
- Radicchio, raw: 204 mg
- Blackberries, raw: 138 mg

- Blueberries, wild, raw: 133 mg

- Tea, green, brewed: 120 mg

- Tea, black, brewed: 119 mg

- Cranberries, raw: 99 mg

- Kale, raw: 93 mg

- Currants, red, raw: 79 mg

- Kumquats, raw: 79 mg

- Blackcurrant, juice: 78 mg

- Tea, white, brewed: 75 mg

- Grapes, Concord, raw: 73 mg

- Arugula, raw: 69 mg

- Mustard greens, raw: 63 mg

- Acai berries, frozen: 62 mg

Foods Containing Caffeine

Caffeine can have mood-altering effects. If you think about the foods that contain caffeine—coffee, black and green teas, and chocolate—you know that these foods have a strong presence and pervasiveness in our society. Depending on the individual, a certain quantity of caffeine may be useful in stimulating the INSIGHT system. In non-users or occasional users of caffeine, low doses (less than 200 mg) can produce a heightened sense of awareness and well-being. However, repeated use may result in ongoing dependency on caffeine.

For most people, coffee is an integral part of early morning and afternoon rituals. When we constantly stimulate our minds, however, we create a need for caffeine. It can become addictive, and even result in low-level withdrawal symptoms like tiredness in the mornings. When we ingest foods consistently and without consciousness, we risk becoming attached to them. With continued use, caffeine can throw your INSIGHT system off balance. Soon after consuming caffeine, you may realize that you are frenetic and unable to concentrate on tasks and simple activities due to the overactive "busy-ness" of your mind.

When heavy caffeine users attempt to eliminate coffee from their bodies for one day or in the course of an elimination diet, they immediately start to develop symptoms, which can be quite severe for some. The body releases caffeine in much the same way as a drug—it shakes, sweats, and aches for days, depending on how long and how much caffeine has been ingested. Eventually, it shifts back to its original state. Most people notice that, once they give up the "need" for caffeine, they feel less anxious.

Of course, on the flip side, caffeine-containing foods can be quite conducive to quick thinking and mental organization when used in their proper context. Remember that it is important to listen to your body's needs on a daily basis so that you can provide it with the proper fuel for its activities.

Cocoa

Cocoa has the potential to change your mood, as it contains several compounds that alter brain neurochemistry in ways that give you that comforting "I'm in love" feeling. Adding milk or sugar to it to create chocolate may alter those brain effects. Many turn to chocolate to soothe their emotions. However, researchers Macdiarmid and Hetherington revealed that eating chocolate for emotional reasons only causes negative emotions. On a pure food-science level, there is much research touting the benefits of chocolate. In addition to the caffeine, cocoa in its pure form contains relatively high amounts of antioxidants known as flavonoids, which can open up our blood vessels. It has been suggested by some researchers that, due to these compounds, cocoa may be beneficial for the heart, and a small daily intake of dark chocolate may lead to decreased blood pressure.

It may prove difficult to substitute other foods for a chocolate craving. There is something uniquely different about chocolate. In a study by researchers Michener and Rozin at the University of Pennsylvania, subjects were given capsules containing the therapeutic, healthy actives in chocolate. Others were given a white chocolate bar that contained none of the actives normally found in cocoa. A third group was given a milk chocolate bar. The group given the milk chocolate bar had reduced cravings compared to all the other groups. Therefore, it's not necessarily the healthy actives that your body craves. There is perhaps a combined effect of the sensory input of the chocolate (slightly bittersweet, smooth texture) combined with the actives that makes people love it.

Spices

You likely have a pharmacy in your kitchen right now, in the form of your spice rack. Using spices is like having a treasure trove of healing plants and herbs at your fingertips, much like dietary supplements. Spices are pungent materials, needed only in small amounts to have a strong flavoring effect. Moreover, many of these botanicals are so potent that they also have medicinal properties. For example, curry powder has strong antioxidant activity and studies show that eating it can help with cognition. In fact, the curcuminoid compounds that are in turmeric, one of the main spices in curry powder, have been shown to have wide-ranging positive effects on inflammation and oxidative stress. Include a variety of spices in your meals so you get a variety of phytochemicals to heal your whole, rainbow self.

Some spices do well in combination with each other. For example, black pepper and turmeric do better together than by themselves. Black pepper enhances the absorption and activity of the curcuminoids in the turmeric. Also, these spices can ward off some of the toxic compounds that form when cooking. Some studies suggest that hamburger meat produces fewer cancer-causing chemicals in the presence of spices like turmeric and rosemary. Some supplements, like fish oil, tend to have a little bit of rosemary in the oil to help preserve it from damage caused by exposure to oxygen. I believe that part of the medicinal impact of the Mediterranean diet may be because of its copious but subtle use of spices in meals.

Here are some spices that help support the INSIGHT system:

Allspice
Anise
Basil
Caraway
Cardamom
Chili powder
Coriander
Cumin

Curry
Dill
Fennel
Fenugreek
Ginger
Horseradish
Mint
Nutmeg
Pepper
Sage
Turmeric
Wasabi

As a nutritionist, I can't speak enough about the advantages of regularly using spices in cooking, as they are important for decreasing inflammation, aiding in healthy digestion, and promoting detoxification. Spices are high-potency sources of plant compounds that fight oxidation and inflammation—the processes underlying disease. In fact, cultures that regularly use a variety of spices have typically been found to be healthier. For example, India has had historically lower rates of dementia, possibly due to the use of curry in cooking. In the Mediterranean region—Greece, Italy, and Spain—spices are integral to meal preparation. Therefore, perhaps it is no coincidence that there are numerous proclaimed benefits to eating dishes from this region.

Three spices that belong in every kitchen are cinnamon, rosemary, and turmeric.

Cinnamon—Beloved Sugar Balancer

This much-beloved spice is used in cuisines around the world. Derived from the bark of a tropical evergreen tree, cinnamon was considered sacred in ancient history. In the United States and Europe, cinnamon is most popular in sweet dishes like apple pie.

Indian and Chinese systems of medicine have embraced cinnamon as a medicine for centuries. In Ayurveda, it is used for respiratory ailments, stomach upset, muscle spasms, and diabetes. In TCM, it is used for its "warming" qualities in respiratory ailments and muscle aches. Cinnamon aids those with type-2 diabetes, because it has both short-term and long-term blood-sugar control properties. Topically, cinnamon is used in suntan lotions, nasal sprays, mouthwashes, gargles, toothpaste, and as a counterirritant in liniments for its wound-healing, anti-microbial, and anti-fungal properties.

Try putting a cinnamon quill in beef or vegetarian stews or in lentil soup for that extra something special. You can also mix cinnamon with mint and parsley in ground beef for burgers or meatloaf, or add it into rice pilaf. It also makes a yummy spiced tea by putting a quart of brewed black tea in a pot with two cups of apple juice. Gently simmer with a sliced lemon and two cinnamon sticks for ten minutes.

Rosemary—The Queen of Flavor

Popular in Mediterranean regions, rosemary thrives in dry, sunny, sandy scrublands near the sea. The word originated from "robe of Mary" in the Christian tradition and eventually morphed into "rosemary." In pre-modern Europe, the French burned rosemary and juniper berries in hospitals to purify the air and prevent disease.

Rosemary has been shown to have many health benefits, including being anti-bacterial, anti-viral, anti-inflammatory, and antioxidant. Research also shows that rosemary aids in dermatitis, memory, cancer, cirrhosis, blood clots, stroke, arthritis, diabetes, ulcers, urinary tract infections (UTIs), and depression.

Rosemary is a hardy spice with a strong flavor that cooks well with meat. Put whole sprigs under roast lamb or place a sprig in the cavity of a whole chicken or fish. Whole sprigs used this way should be removed and discarded. Rosemary does not lose its flavor in long, slow cooking, so it is great in soups and stews. You can finely chop the leaves and add to tomato-based soups, or use it to flavor strong vegetables like Brussels sprouts, cabbage, and eggplant.

Turmeric—The Spice Superstar

Also known as "Indian gold," turmeric has a deep, yellow hue. Commonly used in Indian cuisine, turmeric is a culinary spice and major ingredient in curry powder. It has more than fifty healing actions, including some of these traditional uses:

- As an antacid to soothe digestive problems
- As a powder to speed wound healing and prevent infection (bandages contain turmeric in India)
- As an analgesic to relieve headache
- As a stimulant to improve blood flow
- As a topical paste to clear skin problems
- As a decongestant to clear nasal passages

Turmeric is also known as the "anti-cancer spice," with hundreds of research studies showing how it inhibits the activation of genes that trigger cancer, impedes the spread of tumor cells, hinders the transformation of normal cells into cancer cells, and kills cells that mutate into cancer.

You can easily use more turmeric in the kitchen by adding it to your stir-fries, meats, poultry, or fish recipes. It adds a wonderful little something to soups and stews, and can be used in dishes with cruciferous vegetables for added protection against toxins and to promote healthy metabolic detoxification.

Alcohol

Any substance that alters your consciousness affects and can potentially cloud your inner INSIGHT. For some people, a little alcohol may be helpful and healing, but too much may lead to depressive feelings or shutting down of thought and focus. Sure, we hear a lot about the benefits of the plant bioactives in red wine like resveratrol and polyphenols, but at what cost? Well, some people may say that the effects of the alcohol are fewer because of the healing compounds that are in red wine or hoppy beer. Studies conflict, however, some showing that it may have benefits for cardiovascular health, but some showing it may also lead to cancer or fatty liver or a host of other conditions in a sensitive person. I believe that alcohol intake needs to be personalized to the individual and based on multiple factors such as genetics, environment, and how it is "used," to name a few.

Blue/Purple Foods

Blue/purple foods like grapes, blueberries, and blackberries contain antioxidants known as anthocyanidins. These antioxidants have the greatest "punch" relative to other antioxidants, in terms of their ability to fight damaging free radicals. The anthocyanidin family of compounds acts to protect the brain and nervous system from stress injury. Eating them will help to nourish the INSIGHT system.

Blue/purple vegetables and fruits include:

Blackberries
Blueberries
Boysenberries
Eggplant
Figs
Marionberries
Plums
Purple cabbage
Purple grapes
Purple kale
Purple potato
Raisins

Supplements for Your INSIGHT

As with the FIRE system, you may need to remove foods and substances from your diet to assist your INSIGHT system. To fill the gap, bring in targeted nutrients to help your INSIGHT be as brilliant and remarkable as it can be. In the section below, I talk about supplements that can assist with brain health, particularly neurotransmitter production and improving cognition.

Macronutrient Supplements

As mentioned in other chapters, there are some core macronutrients for our systems of health, and the INSIGHT is no exception. In this section, I will discuss the role of amino acids and fatty acids for your INSIGHT.

Amino Acids

Neurotransmitters are either amino acids like glutamic acid and glycine or made from amino acids—for example, serotonin is made from tryptophan, while dopamine, epinephrine, and norepinephrine are all synthesized from tyrosine. The amino acid methionine combines with ATP to make S-adenosylmethionine (SAM), a compound used to facilitate neurotransmitter production. As a result, it is important to incorporate healthy complete protein sources in the diet for the broad array of essential amino acids that they provide. These amino acids help to balance brain activity through their "excitatory" and "inhibitory" effects.

Essential Fatty Acids

Long-chain essential fats, particularly those from the omega-3 family, are needed for the brain and eyes. Two fatty acids from fish are particularly important: eicosapentaenoic acid (EPA) and docosahexaenoic acid (DHA). EPA supplementation of 1 g twice daily may improve depression, uplift mood, and provide positive changes in personality like reduced aggression. For schizophrenia, 1–3 g in divided doses as EPA or as ethyl-EPA (a particular form of EPA) may be helpful in addition to existing treatment. One g EPA as ethyl-EPA has been recommended for treatment of borderline personality disorder.

The other essential long-chain omega-3, DHA, is found in high concentrations in brain matter (about one-third of the brain is DHA). Infants fed breast milk containing higher levels of essential fat relative to infants fed formula tend to have better cognitive outcomes in the long term. DHA may reduce the risk of age-related macular degeneration, improve attention deficit hyperactivity disorder, and enhance night vision. For infant brain development, 200 mg DHA daily has been recommended for pregnant women, while for night vision, 480 mg DHA has been used.

Both EPA and DHA should be taken with meals. They may interfere with the activity of anticoagulant drugs and promote internal bleeding. Therefore, do not use during pre- or post-surgery.

Vitamins and Minerals

As you may imagine, there can be several roles for vitamins and minerals to play in promoting brain health. In this section, I discuss a few that I think are essential for your INSIGHT.

Vitamin A

Vitamin A (retinol) is required for healthy vision. In vitamin A deficiency, night blindness can occur and eventually progress to complete loss of vision if left untreated. Vitamin A supplements are often taken for improving vision, and for eye diseases like age-related macular degeneration, glaucoma, and cataracts. Note that beta-carotene, which I discuss in chapter 6, is known to convert to vitamin A, although the efficiency of that conversion is different for everyone. See chapter 5 for more details.

Vitamin B6

This vitamin serves as a cofactor for enzymes that convert L-tryptophan to serotonin, and L-tyrosine to norepinephrine. Thus, deficiency may result in depressive symptoms or mood changes. It may play a role in psychiatric disorders and related conditions like Alzheimer's disease, hyperactivity, learning disabilities, and anxiety. Doses of up to 100 mg daily may be helpful in treating premenstrual depression. See chapter 7 for more details.

Vitamin B9

This vitamin is commonly referred to as folic acid. Folate deficiency symptoms that pertain to the INSIGHT system include depression, insomnia, forgetfulness, irritability, and anxiety. There seems to be a relationship between high homocysteine levels and depression. Doses of 800 mcg daily in addition to dietary intake have been shown to reduce levels of homocysteine in the blood substantially. See chapter 5 for more details.

Vitamin B12

Supplementation with vitamin B12 is used for memory loss, sleep disorders, Alzheimer's disease, depression, and psychiatric disorders. Deficiency can lead to cognitive impairment, and personality and mood disorders. Daily oral doses of 2–5 mg cyanocobalamin may be needed to treat deficiency, especially in those who are not able to absorb this vitamin from food or who do not eat vitamin B12-rich foods (e.g., vegetarians). See chapter 5 for more details.

Vitamin C

This water-soluble vitamin (ascorbic acid) plays a crucial role in the metabolism of tyrosine (which converts to dopamine), and as a cofactor in the synthesis of norepinephrine, dopamine, and tryptophan. Psychiatric symptoms related to depression, mania, and paranoia have been shown to improve in patients taking 1 g of ascorbic acid. Individuals with schizophrenia have benefited from vitamin C supplementation, either alone or together with omega-3 fatty acids and vitamin E. See chapter 5 for more details.

Vitamin D

Depressive symptoms and impaired cognitive ability, particularly in the elderly, have been shown to be associated with low vitamin D levels. High doses of vitamin D given to depressed overweight and obese individuals improves depressive symptoms. See chapter 11 for more details.

Magnesium

Magnesium deficiency can cause poor attention, memory loss, restlessness, insomnia, tics, and dizziness. Low levels of magnesium have been reported in depressed individuals. Animal studies have shown that magnesium can act as an anti-depressant and anti-anxiety agent. It is also used to treat premenstrual mood changes and sleep disturbances associated with aging. Typical dose is 125–300 mg daily with meals and at bedtime to help with depression. Magnesium supplementation has also been used to prevent migraine headaches at 600 mg daily. See chapter 8 for more details.

Neurotransmitter Support

Neurotransmitter messengers, traveling from synapse to synapse, form a bridge of communication within the brain. Each neurotransmitter has its role, from being excitatory to calming, or overseeing mood, thought, memory, or cognition. In some cases, we may not have enough of the raw material—individual amino acids—used to make neurotransmitters. Other imbalances can involve not having adequate vitamins or minerals like vitamin C to support the conversion of an amino acid to a neurotransmitter. When neurotransmitters are balanced, the INSIGHT system is perfectly aligned!

5-Hydroxytryptophan (5-HTP)

5-HTP is made in the body from the amino acid L-tryptophan, and is subsequently converted to serotonin. Supplementation with 5-HTP can lead to increased synthesis of serotonin, which is the reason for its use to treat sleep disorders, depression, anxiety, and headaches. Safety is controversial, as there remains a concern as to whether it can cause eosinophilia myalgia syndrome due to the presence of contaminants. Side effects may include gastrointestinal complaints. Do not combine with drugs that alter levels of serotonin. Use under the supervision of a qualified healthcare professional. Doses of 150–300 mg daily have been used for depression.

Acetyl-L-Carnitine

Acetyl-L-carnitine, derived from animal foods like meat and dairy products, is structurally related to the neurotransmitter acetylcholine. It contributes chemical groups to the formation of acetylcholine and promotes its release. Supplementation of acetyl-L-carnitine may be useful in Alzheimer's disease (2–3 g divided into two to three doses daily). It is generally well-tolerated, but gastrointestinal upset and agitation may be experienced by some individuals. This supplement interacts with anticoagulant drugs.

Choline

Choline is a precursor for the neurotransmitter acetylcholine. It is also found as part of the cell membrane phospholipid phosphatidylcholine, which is found within the brain matter. See chapter 7 for more details.

Inositol

Like choline, inositol is incorporated into a phospholipid structure (specifically, phosphatidylinositol) found within all cells in the body, but particularly in the brain. Supplementation with myo-inositol has been used for a variety of conditions. For the INSIGHT system, its effects are most important for its role in aiding the function of neurotransmitter receptors and assisting in regulating neurotransmitter release. Furthermore, it may improve obsessive compulsive disorder, panic disorder, and depression. Although generally well-tolerated, it may cause nausea, fatigue, headaches, and dizziness in some individuals. Certain drugs, like lithium, carbamazepine (Tegretol), and calproic acid, can cause lower levels of inositol in the brain. Doses for different conditions include 12 g daily for depression, 12–18 g daily for panic disorder, and 6 g daily for lithium-induced psoriasis.

St. John's Wort

This plant (*Hypericum perforatum*), typically the flower portion, is used for its anti-depressant activity through its ability to influence levels of neurotransmitters. Use caution when taking in conjunction with medications, as it induces several enzymes that metabolize drugs. Consult a healthcare professional as to whether this botanical should be taken with other medications you are taking. Side effects include insomnia, vivid dreams, restlessness, irritability, dizziness, headache, sensitivity to light, and gastrointestinal upset. If taking other supplements that influence neurotransmitter activity, note that this botanical may produce an additive effect. St. John's wort standardized to 0.3 percent hypericin has been used at a dose of 300 mg three times daily for mild to moderate depression.

Sleep Support

Sleep provides an opportunity for a recharge of the INSIGHT system, allowing it to process visual stimuli, thoughts, situations, and events over a lifetime or during a day. Without good quality and quantity of sleep, you become depleted and are left unable to focus, concentrate, think clearly, or even regulate your moods. Specific supplements can assist you in sleeping well and dreaming. Dreams are a window into inner intuitive dimensions. To help heal this part of your spectrum, log your dreams in a journal and reflect on their potential symbolism and meaning.

Hops

Hop cones contain a volatile oil that may have sedative properties. Traditionally, the hop plant (*Humulus lupulus*) has been used to treat anxiety, insomnia, and sleep disorders, often in conjunction with other therapies, since the effects of hops are relatively mild. Side effects include depression, confusion, memory changes, hallucinations, and seizures. Do not use with alcohol or with supplements or drugs that have sedative properties. Use of hops with hormone-sensitive cancers is not advised, since hops have estrogenic properties.

Lemon Balm

The leaf and leaf oil of lemon balm (*Melissa officinalis*) induce calming and sedative effects. Oral extracts (and oils in aromatherapy) are used for treating anxiety, insomnia, restlessness, agitation in Alzheimer's disease, and attention deficit hyperactivity disorder. Side effects include gastrointestinal complaints, dizziness, and wheezing. Additive effects may occur when taken with other supplements or drugs with sedative or depressant effects.

Melatonin

Melatonin is a hormone made and secreted by the pineal gland that plays a role in sleep patterns and circadian rhythm. Its secretion is regulated by light-dark cycles. Melatonin can be taken as a dietary supplement for insomnia, jet lag, circadian rhythm disorders, Alzheimer's disease, depression, sleep-wake cycle disturbances, and cluster headaches. It is generally well-tolerated, but can result in daytime drowsiness, headache, dizziness, and even seizures in some people. Do not operate machinery for four to five hours after taking melatonin. Taking melatonin with anticoagulant and sedative drugs may potentiate their effects. Avoid melatonin from animal sources (for example, animal-sourced pineal gland material) due to the potential for contaminants. Doses of 0.3–3 mg at bedtime have been used for insomnia, and up to 9 mg for sleep disturbances in Alzheimer's disease.

Passionflower

This herb (*Passiflora incarnata*) has been used for insomnia and anxiety. Side effects include dizziness, confusion, sedation, and ataxia (incoordination of muscle movements). This botanical may interact with supplements and drugs that have sedative properties.

Valerian Root

The root and rhizome of this plant (*Valeriana officinalis*) have sedative, hypnotic, anti-anxiety, and anti-depressive effects. It has been used traditionally for insomnia, improving time to sleep onset and sleep quality, as well as anxiety, restlessness, depression, and attention deficit hyperactivity disorder. Valerian is often combined with other sedative herbs like hops. Side effects include headache, excitability, insomnia, cardiac disturbance, gastric complaints, vivid dreams, and morning drowsiness. There are also reports that it caused liver toxicity. The long-term effects of valerian on liver function remain unknown. Exercise caution if combining valerian with other herbs or drugs that have sedative effects. Do not use with alcohol, Xanax, benzodiazepines, or CNS depressants. Since it may influence the metabolism of a number of drugs, use under the supervision of a qualified healthcare professional. A 600 mg dose of valerian extract has shown favorable outcome when given thirty minutes before bedtime to insomniacs for twenty-eight days.

Eye Support

The INSIGHT system is responsible for vision—not just the ability to see the outside world (our eyes), but also inner vision and perception of what is illusion and what is truth. Nutrients like vitamin A and potent colored pigments like lutein, zeaxanthin, and bilberry can provide the eyes with healing support. If you are experiencing visual problems, ask yourself these questions: What am I not willing to see? What is clouding my vision?

Bilberry Fruit Extract

In addition to its effects on the circulation of blood and on blood-sugar lowering, the high concentration of purple pigments (anthocyanidins) contained within bilberry fruit (*Vaccinium myrtillus*) may be useful for eye afflictions like night vision, low visual acuity, cataracts, and retinal conditions, particularly those related to diabetes. Please work with a qualified healthcare provider if you wish to supplement with bilberry and you are diabetic.

Lutein and Zeaxanthin

This yellow-pigmented carotenoid is found in green-yellow vegetables like broccoli, spinach, and kale. It typically occurs together with another carotenoid, zeaxanthin. Both lutein and zeaxanthin are highly concentrated in the human macula and retina. It is thought that they function as antioxidants, protecting the fragile eye tissue from light damage. In population studies, people with a high dietary intake of lutein have decreased risk for developing severe cataracts and age-related macular degeneration (AMD). Lutein supplements (10–30 mg) have been shown to benefit people with AMD, cataracts, and retinal disorders.

Cognition Support

The INSIGHT system supports the faculty of cognition by piecing together all input and synthesizing it into thought. Our ability to focus, learn, and retain information is determined by the workings of the brain. If our minds are clear and uncluttered, we can concentrate more effectively. In addition to EPA and DHA, there are some other botanicals and nutrients that can be helpful in keeping the mind sharp and focused, as well as some mind-body therapies that are useful. Meditation may also be helpful for this purpose. Strengthen your mind through affirmations and mantras, and by keeping it elastic through a variety of mental activities.

Brahmi

This Ayurvedic herb (*Bacopa monnieri*) is commonly used to enhance learning and memory, relieve anxiety, and reduce the symptoms of attention deficit hyperactivity disorder. The leaf, which contains the actives bacosides A and B, may modulate acetylcholine release, a neurotransmitter important in memory. A dose of 300 mg brahmi extract improved verbal learning, memory, and information processing in healthy people.

Gotu Kola

Gotu kola (*Centella asiatica*) has been used in traditional medicine for reducing anxiety and depression, and for increasing memory and intelligence. It may work by influencing GABA receptors in the brain. Through its ability to improve blood circulation, it may also stimulate brain function. Side effects may include gastrointestinal complaints, nausea, drowsiness, and liver toxicity (elevated liver enzymes). Do not use with herbs, supplements, or drugs that affect the liver or that have sedative properties. A recent study showed that 750 mg of a gotu kola plant extract for two months positively affected mood and cognition in an elderly population.

L-Theanine

This amino acid is found in low levels (1–3 percent) in green tea. It has been shown to impact brain function. Studies using human electroencephalographs (EEG, a device used to measure the electrical activity of the brain) have shown that as little as 50 mg of L-theanine can promote the frequency of alpha waves in the brain—waves that relax the mind without drowsiness. Supplementation with L-theanine has been used for anxiety, Alzheimer's disease, and improving cognition. Use with caution if taking together with supplements or drugs that lower blood pressure, as it is thought that L-theanine can enhance these effects. For improving cognition (specifically, the ability to sustain attention to a mental task), 250 mg daily has been found to have favorable effects. Studies have demonstrated that, when L-theanine (100 mg) is combined with caffeine (50 mg), there is significant improvement in the speed and accuracy of cognitive tasks.

Phosphatidylserine

One of the most abundant phospholipids (a type of fat) in the brain, phosphatidylserine has been used for Alzheimer's disease, dementia, mental function decline, attention deficit hyperactivity disorder, and depression. It has been shown in studies to improve attention, verbal fluency, and memory in people with age-associated cognitive decline, and to improve cognition and behavior in Alzheimer's disease. Side effects include gastrointestinal complaints and insomnia. Avoid animal-derived sources of phosphatidylserine due to the risk for contamination. Vegetable forms like soy-sourced phosphatidylserine are recommended if you do not have a soy allergy. Supplementation with phosphatidylserine may interact with all drugs that modify the levels or action of acetylcholine in the brain. Typical dose is 100 mg three times daily for Alzheimer's disease, dementia, or aging adults with memory impairment.

CHAPTER 11

THE WHITE SPIRIT

The true way to be humble is not to stoop until you are smaller than yourself, but to stand at your real height against some higher nature that will show you what the real smallness of your greatness is.

Phillips Brooks

KEY WORDS FOR THE SPIRIT: connection, divinity, infinite, interconnectedness, purity, purpose, radiance, soul, source, spirit, spirituality, unity, universe, universal truth, white

The SPIRIT system holds the entry way for universal awareness to enlighten our being. It contains our beliefs about something greater than ourselves. I like to define "spirituality" as feeling the interconnectedness of life and having a deep understanding of the "why" of living. Spirituality need not adhere to any particular text or practices. It can simply be rolled into the way in which we live life—smiling at a stranger on the street, sharing lunch with a friend, or calling a relative just to say hello. Spirituality is a call to emphasize our relationship with all of life. Our SPIRIT systems allow us to feel a sense of awe and wonder at the experience of living. As Stephen Covey has said: "We are spiritual beings living in earthly bodies."

The SPIRIT and Your Body

We are physical beings, but we are also composed of things we can't see, like EMFs or even the non-visible spray of light we may give off, called biophotonic emission by certain scientists. At the level of the SPIRIT system, we are quantum particles. This system of health is reserved for the non-physical, non-visible parts of us. It represents the electricity of the life force within the body, and can be referred to as *chi*, *qi*, or *prana*. In addition to the electromagnetic force to which we are connected, the SPIRIT system contains the activity of the central nervous system throughout the body. The nervous system's branches and bundles align closely with the non-visible channels of energy that course through our bodies. In TCM, these networks are known as energy meridians.

With the SPIRIT system, we turn our attention to the power of the smallest particle. Within our physiology, these are atoms, protons, neutrons, electrons, and even photons, miniscule particles of light. Light is essential for our good health: sunlight, bright light, ultraviolet light, and colored lights are all healing in the right doses. Recently, we have begun to see the application of light in medicine through technologies like lasers.

The SPIRIT and Eating

How can something so ethereal be connected with something as essential to your physical body as eating? There is definitely a way to make your eating more soul-full. Here are some questions to ask yourself to determine if you are feeding your spiritual being and supporting your SPIRIT system.

Do you make eating a spiritual practice?

The highest expression of the spirit as it relates to foods and eating is to turn the entire experience into a means of "in-*light*enment," or a spiritual practice. When you have an intention to infuse sacredness into every moment of the eating event, you reap the miracle of the moments in which you are eating. Theology professor Kelton Cobb captured this idea best in the following quote:

> The table, the trough, has God's fingerprints all over it. We participate in a mystery whenever we eat food. Indeed, every meal is sacramental. Through eating, death is resurrected into life. Dead fish, dead figs, and dead cornflakes are transformed into the living tissue of our bodies. . . . That is an event I would call sacred—a holy occurrence.

What and how you choose to eat says something about your relationship to your spirit. Do you eat in a hurried manner, trying to find a shortcut to a divine or holy experience? Are you stuffing your mouth, attempting to fill the emptiness within due to a lack of connection with all of life? Do you numb and distract yourself with foods rather than look at the deeper, soul-full issues in your life? Do you feel interconnected to all life?

I celebrate myself and sing myself;

And what I assume you shall assume;

For every atom belonging to me, as good belongs to you.

Walt Whitman, *Leaves of Grass*

Do you pray or meditate at meals?

We discussed gratitude when we delved into the LOVE system. Gratitude for foods helps us to center ourselves in respect for the eating process and all that is involved in it, from beginning to end. Prayer or meditation further anchors your heartfelt gratitude in divinity and something greater than yourself. Besides the spoken word, prayer may be received in the form of an action, like bowing your head or putting your hands together.

When you pray over a meal, you recognize the sacredness in the entire offering. A spiritual mentor of mine once commented: "Prayer is us talking to God. Intuition is God talking to us."

Have you released excessive attachments to food?

When you operate in fear mode, you can become fixated on survival, and "having enough." Linda described how she never felt at peace unless she knew where her next meal was coming from. She struggled with issues of abundance. When you come from a place of lack all the time, you eat out of a need to "be filled," rather than finding the source of fulfillment within. Instead, trust that you will have enough if you rely on the strength of your inner spirit to guide you.

Do you purify your body through fasting?

Since your spirit is not physical, it does not require food. It feeds off of spiritual morsels of prayer and divine inspiration. When you fast, you cast off the physical energy and residue that prevent you from having a clean, clear spirit. You replace the physical nourishment with spiritual sustenance.

Most religious and spiritual traditions practice fasting, in which certain foods are omitted or included. For example, the Islamic tradition of Ramadan is a forty-day fast during which no food is eaten before sundown. Similarly, the Roman Catholic season of Lent involves eating fish on Fridays. It is a common practice during Lent to give up some item—often a food item.

Releasing yourself in some degree from the practice of eating may allow your body's needs to be suspended temporarily so that the needs of the spirit may be addressed. Of course, due to health reasons, some individuals may not be able to fast, or perhaps should do so under the supervision of a trained medical professional. There are many manifestations of fasting. For example, a fast may be as simple as skipping lunch on Sundays, or it may be several days of replacing all solid food with fresh squeezed juices.

Do you try to "go simple"?

Because of its non-physical nature, your spirit doesn't need as much involvement with physical activities like meal selection and preparation. With the SPIRIT system, go "simple." When it comes to eating, you can bring the element of simplicity to biting into a piece of fresh fruit, picking a vegetable from the garden, or taking a precious sip from a glass of pure water. Whole foods in their natural form are most fitting for the SPIRIT system.

In addition to eating simple foods, try eating without much fuss. Don Gerrard has written a book called *One Bowl* that introduces the concept of always eating from the same bowl. By deliberately focusing your intention on a particular eating vessel, you can concentrate it with healing and loving thoughts and actions.

Are you choosing pure, unadulterated foods?

Foods that are pure keep the metabolic machinery of the physical body flowing. Pure foods are plants that are grown in the absence of pesticides, herbicides, and insecticides, with their DNA left intact (not genetically modified). Heirloom seeds and plants are great for this purpose. For animal foods to be considered pure, they must be fed high-quality, non-GMO feed, be free to range, and not be injected with unnecessary hormones or antibiotics. It is ideal if both plants and animals are cultivated in a loving environment, in accordance with natural principles.

In contrast, try to avoid artificial, synthetic foods like artificial sweeteners, soft drinks, partially hydrogenated (trans) fat, and GMO foods.

Eating Activities for the SPIRIT

1. Before eating, try "bathing" your food in the brilliance of sunlight. Allow your plate full of food to bask in the sun for a couple of minutes.

2. Create a prayer or intention to say before eating.

3. How do you eat? What does this suggest about your spirit?

4. Create or buy a bowl or plate that you use for all your meals. Try using it exclusively for one week. Journal on your experience.

5. Instead of a "mind-full" exercise with food, try a "spirit-full" experience with food. With each bite, imagine unlocking the spirituality that pervades the matrix of the food. How does this connection help to put you in touch with something bigger than yourself?

6. Plan to do a whole-body cleansing program, like the Whole Detox program I created, that you follow based on the needs of your body and soul (see my website for more information).

7. Infuse your food with a meaningful intention before eating.

Foods for Your SPIRIT

We eat light. Every bit of food represents the energy of the sun. After all, foods begin with the sun's rays, which are captured by the chlorophyll within plants. Those plants harness energy and growth with the help of the sun. When we eat plants, or perhaps animals that have eaten plants, we take in the energy of the sun with every bite. The sun helps plants to photosynthesize. It gives us the energy of warmth, and it sets our biological rhythms through our pineal gland, which is part of the SPIRIT system.

Sunlight

Sunlight can permeate your physical being and spark certain cell processes. Ultraviolet light has been shown to activate a vitamin D precursor in the skin to its active form. Vitamin D is used throughout the body for a variety of functions.

Air

Oxygen supports our underlying need for energy. It keeps our being conscious, alive, and invigorated, and fuels energy exchanges within cells. Eastern Indian tradition associates the breath, or *prana*, with the spiritual life force energy. In much the same way, oxygen provides the human organism with the energy it needs to sustain itself.

Certain incense and smudging herbs can be purifying for the SPIRIT system. Herbs such as dried white sage, copal, myrrh, frankincense, and juniper are not meant to be eaten, but are ritually burned in a safe container to create smoke that we inhale through the nostrils.

Detoxification

The SPIRIT system emphasizes the need for purification and clarification. Cleansing is an age-old practice within both spiritual and medical traditions. Over time, it is natural to get a build-up of toxic products in your body from the air you breathe and from the foods you eat. Every season, it is a nourishing practice to undergo a detoxification of your external and internal environment to purify your body and clarify your mind. When you detoxify, it is like pushing an internal reset button.

Of course, there are many ways to do a detoxification. Some people like juicing, others consume only water, some turn to nutritional support like vitamins and minerals. Using nutritional support may be optimal, as supplementation can provide you with necessary nutrients to assist in the disposal of what you no longer need. In conjunction with a physical detoxification, I have people participate in an emotional, mental, and spiritual detoxification as well. (This is called Whole Detox, which is the title of one of my other books). During this time, the focus is on letting go of unnecessary emotional patterns, thoughts, and beliefs.

You can also transition to a more rigorous detoxification program by eating "light," or smaller portions. Caloric restriction in animals has been shown to result in increased lifespan. By reducing your energy input through physical matter, you create more balance with the non-physical spirit. Fewer toxins are formed and you are rewarded with a longer life.

In the table below, you'll find some ideas as to what you can do to address toxins from each system of health. For a more comprehensive program, read my book, *Whole Detox*.

TABLE 2. A WHOLE-SELF, FULL-SPECTRUM APPROACH TO DETOXIFICATION

Week	System of Health	Modalities	Release/Replace
1	ROOT	Increased fiber	Release fear and outdated ancestral patterns that no longer serve you; replace with safety and trust
2	FLOW	Increased water intake, sweating through sauna (especially steam sauna), use of salt baths	Release blocks in creative flow and emotions; replace with embracing personal expression
3	FIRE	Movement of any type, dry sauna, full-body massage	Release unnecessary control, disempowered thoughts, and frustration; replace with courage and personal power
4	LOVE	Listening to music, singing, deep breathing	Release hatred and bitterness; replace with compassion and love
5	TRUTH	Examine and extract toxic language in your speech	Release deception and artificiality; replace with truth and authenticity
6	INSIGHT	Nourishing sleep, dream analysis	Release overthinking and illusion; replace with detachment and intuition
7	SPIRIT	Meditation, silence, stillness	Release attachment to food and body; replace with connection to all of life and unity

White Foods

When I grew up in the 1970s, my mom used to say to me: "The whiter the bread, the quicker you're dead." If we look at our current food supply, there are several foods that are "white" and unhealthy because they've been stripped of nutrients: table sugar, flour, rice, pasta, bread, marshmallows, and crackers. In all these cases, white is not considered a healing color of purity and detoxification—in fact, just the opposite!

There are, however, some nutritious, white-colored foods. And when I refer to the colors of foods—yellow, orange, green, blue, purple, and red—I also include "white" in that list. Our human vision may not pick up all the colorless phytonutrients, but they are present and extremely valuable, nonetheless!

Here are some examples of healthy white foods and some tips for their use.

Cauliflower

Cauliflower is one of the many cruciferous vegetables that can assist in healthy detoxification processes in the liver. It is more than half as potent as the "detox superstars," broccoli and kale. Eating cauliflower is a good way to add some variety to your cruciferous vegetable intake. A study by Kirsh, et al. (2007) found: "High intake of cruciferous vegetables, including broccoli and cauliflower, may be associated with reduced risk of aggressive prostate cancer, particularly extraprostatic disease." Cauliflower has a low glycemic index of 15–30. One of my favorite ways to prepare it is to sauté the florets briefly in extra-virgin olive oil and spices and serve warm. A newer trend is to make a "cauliflower rice," which involves shredding the cauliflower into smaller rice-sized particles and gently steaming and stir-frying.

Coconut Milk and Oil

My recipes emphasize coconut oil and coconut milk, primarily because they contain short- and medium-chain fats that are helpful for healing the gut, and are quickly burned as fuel by the liver. Coconut products have a reputation for their anti-microbial and anti-viral effects. One recent study surprisingly showed that an extra-virgin coconut oil-containing diet decreased waist size and increased good cholesterol in people with coronary artery disease. My word of caution is: "Don't overdo it." I have observed that, as a food-loving culture, we become enamored with what I call "nutritional darlings." We tend to believe that, if a little is good, a lot is better. My approach with milk substitutes and oils is to use a variety of them on a daily basis.

Garlic

Garlic has many medicinal uses, from lowering cholesterol to balancing blood sugar to helping with heart health and blood pressure. When it comes to detox, its sulfur and selenium content come in handy for assisting liver enzymes to remove toxins. Let raw garlic sit after cutting it to maximize the production of protective antioxidants.

Onions

These gorgeous white orbs are healing and helpful for blood sugar, heart health, and detox. They contain at least twenty-five different plant compounds called flavonoids, including one of the most popular ones known as quercetin, a potent antioxidant. Red onions tend to contain just a bit more of the flavonol phytonutrients than yellow onions, although there is some variability based on where the onions are grown. Most of those phytonutrients are right below the skin, so do not overpeel your onions! Onions have a very low glycemic index of 10–15.

Turnips and Parsnips

Turnips have a low glycemic index in raw form, and a high one when cooked. Parsnips, on the other hand, have only a medium-to-high glycemic index when cooked. They are both suited for use in stews and soups, as both provide great opportunities to increase fiber intake, along with a complex array of different plant nutrients that protect the body from oxidative stress damage. Do not overcook them, however, because they will become mushy and higher in glycemic impact. If you want to, you can shred them into your salads as a tasty touch!

Supplements for Your SPIRIT

While your SPIRIT may not need much in the way of physical substances, there are some supplements you can bring in for greater bodily purification, as well as to fine-tune your ultra-fine nervous system.

Macronutrients for Purity

Purification is pivotal for the SPIRIT system, as it assists the body in the removal of toxins. This process may involve the assistance of other body tissues like the skin (the ROOT system), the extracellular matrix, kidneys, and colon (the FLOW system), the liver and small intestine (the FIRE system), and the lungs (the LOVE system).

Detoxification programs that focus on using various modalities, including supplements, may be effective for keeping the body collective harmonized and resonating. Examples of these supplements include:

- Insoluble and soluble fiber for trapping toxins in the gut and carrying them out of the body (see chapter 6)

- Liver support to optimize the internal transformation of toxic substances and their eventual excretion (see chapter 7)

- Alkalizing minerals like magnesium and potassium to assist the kidneys in efficiently releasing toxins in the urine.

Hypoallergenic Powders for Detoxification

These powdered supplements are devoid of the top eight allergens—milk, eggs, peanuts, tree nuts, fish, shellfish, soy, and wheat. They are often made from rice, since it is considered to be hypo-allergenic for most people, and expressly address the detoxification of the body by cleansing the liver or the gut. They are helpful for all systems of health.

Essential Fatty Acids

The central nervous system is highly enriched in the essential omega-6 and omega-3 fats. As seen in chapters 6 and 10, these important fats are integrated throughout the body and are needed for it to function normally. For the SPIRIT system, adequate intake of these fats is needed for the development of nerve cells in the fetus.

Omega-3 Fatty Acids

Omega-3 fats, particularly the long-chain fats from fish and algae, EPA and DHA (see chapters 6 and 10), are important for nerve-cell membrane composition and for healthy blood flow to nerve cells. Diabetics with neuropathy who took 1800 mg EPA for forty-eight weeks experienced reduced coldness and numbness and better nerve symptoms. Compared with olive oil, fish oil (comprised of both EPA and DHA) administration resulted in nerve regeneration in diabetic rats. EPA and DHA supplementation holds promise for those with chronic nerve degeneration conditions, and may also be beneficial in acute nerve injuries.

Omega-6 Fatty Acids

The omega-6 fat gamma linolenic acid (GLA) is important for nerve membrane structure. It is conceivable that deficiency or reduced levels of omega-6 may lead to neuropathy. The human studies investigating GLA supplementation for diabetic neuropathy showed that 360–480 mg GLA for six months to a year resulted in better nerve function. Animal studies with diabetic rats showed that GLA improved nerve health and nerve blood flow.

Vitamins and Minerals

To ensure the smooth and streamlined function of your SPIRIT, some vitamins and minerals are essential for detoxification and nervous-system function.

Multivitamins

Multivitamins contain a broad spectrum of nutritional substances for the entire body, and are excellent for balancing and integrating the whole being. Of course, they are not meant to take the place of a balanced diet. Their use is to supply the body with small amounts of nutrients that will subtly supplement any shortcomings of the diet based on day-to-day variation. With added stress because of the polluted and toxic environment in which we live, it is essential to have added "nutritional insurance." Since a multivitamin is often taken on a daily basis, it should be free of unessential preservatives, fat, dyes, and sweeteners like sucralose, any of the FD&C colors, hydrogenated oil, and BHT. If you have an allergy to corn, avoid multivitamins that contain corn starch or maltodextrin (often corn-derived).

Vitamin B1

Vitamin B1, or thiamin, deficiency typically results in neurological symptoms. Chronic alcoholic use can result in thiamin deficiency and, ultimately, to neuropathy. The fat-soluble form of thiamin, called benfotiamine, has been touted as the preferred compound (relative to its water-soluble form) for promoting nerve-cell health in neuropathic conditions. However, results from studies indicated mixed findings. Some evidence suggests that benfotiamine may be helpful in relieving pain in individuals with peripheral neuropathy when taken at 400 mg daily (two 50 mg tablets taken four times throughout the day). Benfotiamine may work synergistically with a B-vitamin complex. See chapter 7 for more details.

Vitamin B6

This essential B vitamin has a unique relationship with neuropathies: its deficiency is associated with the development of peripheral neuropathy (neuropathy in the extremities), while high doses (1–5 g daily) may *cause* peripheral neuropathy. See chapter 7 for more details.

Vitamin B7

Deficiency of vitamin B7, or biotin, is relatively rare, but it can occur with malabsorption syndromes, pregnancy, long-term parenteral nutrition, and diabetes. It can lead to neurological symptoms like tingling or prickling sensations, or numbness (a condition referred to as paresthesia). Lower levels of biotin have been found in the cerebrospinal fluid (fluid in the spinal column) and blood of people with multiple sclerosis and epilepsy compared to people without these conditions. In a small study with people on dialysis that had peripheral neuropathy, 10 mg of biotin taken in divided doses throughout the day for one to four years resulted in improved paresthesia, restless legs, and increased ability to walk. See chapter 5 for more details.

Vitamin B12

Vitamin B12 is used as an anti-aging agent and for tremors. Deficiency results in neurological damage, including impairments in the production of myelin (fatty sheath around nerves), and may lead to nerve-cell damage. High levels of neurotoxic inflammatory compounds (called cytokines) and decreased levels of nerve-supporting factors (growth factors) have been found in B12 deficiency. Testing levels of homocysteine in the blood may help to identify those at risk for deficiency. See chapter 5 for more details.

Vitamin C

Vitamin C deficiency can result in nervous-system dysfunction. When administered alone or together with vitamin E, vitamin C can prevent decreased nerve conduction that occurs under cold temperature extremes. Both these vitamins help to reverse age-related neuron changes. See chapter 5 for more details.

Vitamin D

Although the primary function of vitamin D connects most closely with the ROOT system because of its involvement with calcium and bone structure, it also extends to the realm of the SPIRIT system. Vitamin D is derived through sunshine and acts like a hormone, creating alignment within body systems. It may play a role in preventing nerve degeneration and in conditions that involve the nervous and immune systems (e.g., multiple sclerosis). See chapter 5 for more details.

Vitamin E

Vitamin E deficiency (associated with intestinal diseases and malabsorption) may lead to neurological symptoms. When people with diabetic neuropathy were given 900 mg of vitamin E for six months, their nerve function improved more than the group not given vitamin E. It may also help in neurotoxicity caused by chemotherapy. See chapter 6 for more details.

Magnesium

Diabetics are typically lower in magnesium than healthy people. A daily dose of 300 mg to magnesium-deficient type-1 diabetics was able to prevent the progressive worsening of neuropathic symptoms.

Nervous System Support

The SPIRIT system permeates the entire human body through the intricate web of the nervous system. If nerves are damaged or degenerating (neuropathy), they may cause pain, numbness, and tingling sensations. From a physiological perspective, these effects can occur due to chronic diseases like diabetes, exposure to environmental toxins, alcoholism, nutritional deficiencies, or as a side effect of a medication. If you are experiencing these conditions, ask yourself: Where am I experiencing pain in my spirit? Do I feel cut off from or numb to my spiritual nature?

Acetyl-L-Carnitine

Acetyl-L-carnitine assists the SPIRIT system in a variety of ways through its effects on the central nervous system. It can protect nerve cells from damage, promote communication between nerves (neurotransmission), and enhance energy production in nerve cells. It may help the nerve cells to function better when under conditions of low oxygen (hypoxia), as shown in animal studies. Supplementation of acetyl-L-carnitine can be particularly beneficial when coupled with alpha lipoic acid. Individuals with multiple sclerosis who were supplemented with acetyl-L-carnitine had lower levels of reactive, damaging compounds in their cerebrospinal fluid, compared with those with the condition who were not supplemented, or with people with neurological conditions not involving inflammation. Side effects include nausea, vomiting, gastrointestinal complaints, restlessness, and fishy odor of the urine, breath, and sweat. Do not take together with anticoagulants or use in hypothyroidism or in those susceptible to seizures. For diabetic neuropathy, 1500–3000 mg daily in divided doses has been used therapeutically. See chapter 10 for more details.

Alpha Lipoic Acid

Alpha lipoic acid is commonly found in meats and a variety of vegetables. Perhaps due to its role as a lipid antioxidant (protects fat in the body from damage by oxygen), it has been shown to protect nerves from inflammation and toxicity. Oral intake has been helpful for neuropathies in the legs and feet. Side effects may include nausea and skin rash. Avoid use with supplements and drugs that lower blood sugar. Supplementation with alpha lipoic acid may decrease the effectiveness of chemotherapy. At doses of 600–1800 mg daily, symptoms of diabetic neuropathy like burning, pain, numbness, and prickling of feet and legs may be alleviated. See chapter 7 for more details.

Choline

Choline is highly concentrated in nerve tissue. Supplementation of choline during pregnancy may impact the structure of neurons that play a role in the memory in the developing fetus. Additionally, choline may help prevent neural tube defects. See chapter 7 for more details.

Coenzyme Q10

This potent antioxidant may protect against nerve damage produced by lack of oxygen, accumulation of plaque in the arteries, and by injury. Studies have shown that people with early-stage Parkinson's disease may benefit from supplementation of 300–1200 mg daily. See chapter 8 for more details.

Gotu Kola

Gotu kola (*Centella asiatica*) has a reputation as a "spiritual herb" in the Ayurvedic tradition. In addition to its effects on the mind and on blood circulation, it may also have effects on longevity and the healing of nerve cells, as it has been shown to accelerate the repair of damaged nerve cells. Side effects may include gastrointestinal complaints, nausea, drowsiness, and liver toxicity (elevated liver enzymes). Do not use with herbs, supplements, or drugs that affect the liver or that have sedative properties. See chapters 8 and 10 for other uses.

Inositol

Inositol is situated within specific lipids (phospholipids) in nerve cell membranes. Low levels of myo-inositol in nerve cells have been associated with the underlying dysfunction related to diabetic neuropathy. In animal studies, myo-inositol prevented nerve degeneration. In a small human study, nerve myo-inositol levels were lower in people with diabetic neuropathy when compared with those tested without the condition. Finally, in people with normal or abnormal blood-sugar balance, high levels of nerve myo-inositol were connected with better nerve cell health (indicated by increased nerve fiber density). See chapters 6 and 10 for other uses.

Support for Aging

Vitality, as measured by life quality and quantity, belongs to the SPIRIT system. Aiming for mastery of the mind and body has been part of the daily practice of the ancient wise ones. Being able to control bodily functions and, ultimately, the aging process, indicates that the SPIRIT system is in full lotus-like bloom. Of course, a variety of practices can help, like deep breathing (a full acceptance and merging with all of life), yoga (integrating body and mind), and eating pure, clean foods. Including supplements that enhance the overall health of the body (and spirit) is also useful.

Resveratrol

Resveratrol is a natural compound found in the skin of grapes and in the leaf of the grape plant. Many of the health-promoting qualities of red wine are those demonstrated by resveratrol in cell and animal studies—its ability to be anti-inflammatory, to reduce platelet aggregation, to serve as an antioxidant and anti-cancer compound, and to favorably modify fat metabolism. It appears to protect nerve cells from damage and death from inflammation, as shown in cell and animal studies. Newer research in various organisms (from yeast to rodents) suggests that it can activate enzymes in the body (sirtuins) that mimic the effects of caloric restriction, which may decrease aging and the onset of age-related diseases, and aid in lifespan extension. Research is still lacking regarding its ability to prolong lifespan in humans.

If taking resveratrol, note that it acts as a phytoestrogen (see chapter 6) and may potentiate estrogen's effects in the body. Therefore, individuals with hormone-sensitive conditions like breast, uterine, and ovarian cancer, as well as endometriosis and fibroids, should avoid or use under the guidance of a qualified healthcare professional. Do not take together with supplements or drugs that have anticoagulant properties. Resveratrol also has the capacity to influence the metabolism of certain drugs.

CHAPTER 12

HOW TO PERSONALIZE
YOUR RAINBOW DIET

Individuality is only possible if it unfolds from wholeness.

David Bohm

Based on what you have learned about your inner spectrum and and your seven systems of health, you can now create your own personalized eating plan. Again, check with your healthcare practitioner(s) before embarking upon any significant dietary change. These are only ideas for you to consider.

The Quick Three-Day Plan

Once you know in which colors your imbalances reside, focus on those colors in your eating for three consecutive days. For example, if your scores were high for the ROOT and INSIGHT systems, emphasize protein, minerals, insoluble fiber, red-colored foods, spices, cocoa, and blue/purple-colored foods in your diet over a few days to see how you feel. At the end of three days, take the Spectrum Quiz again to get your scores. If you continue to be imbalanced in these areas, allow for a bit more time—about seven days total—of focusing on these systems. Instead of just addressing food, see if you can incorporate some eating strategies as well.

The Seven-Day Plan

Regardless of your Spectrum Quiz scores, you can dedicate one day per week to each of the seven systems of health. For each day, put all your efforts into the colorful foods and the eating practices that correspond to the color of that system. For example, on day one, eat red-colored foods and the foods that correspond to the ROOT system, like protein. You can also engage in some of the ROOT eating practices mentioned in chapter 5. On day two, do the same for the FLOW system. Eat orange-colored foods, with a focus on fat and oil, water, nuts, and seeds. You may even wear orange, and assess whether you are expressing your emotions. On day three, shift your energy to the FIRE system by incorporating yellow-colored, healthy foods. Assess your carbohydrate intake and note your energy levels as you eat specific foods. Continue this pattern through to day seven and the SPIRIT system.

The Seven-Week Plan

Some people tell me they are overwhelmed by all the features of each system and that they really want to "do it right" when it comes to balancing each one. If this sounds like you, you may enjoy really sinking into each system, devoting a week to each one. Start with the ROOT system and work your way through the other six a week at a time. If you have the ability and the inclination, this is a wonderful way to get to know your systems deeply. Doing this practice once a year may suffice for most people. The shorter three-day and seven-day plans can be done more frequently throughout the year.

The Daily Balancing Plan

Maybe you'd just like to notice how all your systems come together on a daily basis. In that case, assess the colors of food you are eating on a daily basis, along with their quality. Examples of this daily spectrum strategy are given in the tables below for reference.

TABLE 3. SAMPLE MENU #1*

Meal	Foods	Systems
Breakfast	Coconut milk smoothie made with mango, hard-boiled egg, expression of gratitude	ROOT, FLOW, LOVE, TRUTH
Snack	Celery and carrot sticks with hummus, black tea	ROOT, FLOW, FIRE, LOVE, TRUTH, INSIGHT
Lunch	Mixed green salad with cherry tomatoes, pine nuts, olives, and cucumbers plus one small cup lentil soup, small glass pomegranate juice, all infused with love	ROOT, FLOW, FIRE, LOVE, TRUTH
Snack	Plain, unsweetened yogurt with mixed berries and ground flaxseed meal	ROOT, FLOW, LOVE, INSIGHT
Dinner	Asian vegetable stir-fry (bamboo shoots, sprouts, snap peas, Chinese eggplant) with chicken, jasmine tea, prayer	ROOT, LOVE, TRUTH, INSIGHT, SPIRIT
Snack	Baked apple with cinnamon	ROOT, FIRE, INSIGHT

* Note that regular eating times feed the FIRE and TRUTH systems; water should be sipped throughout the day to feed the FLOW system.

TABLE 4. SAMPLE MENU #2

Meal	Foods	Systems
Breakfast	Steel-cut oatmeal plus flaxseed meal with coconut milk, walnuts, honey	ROOT, FLOW, FIRE
Snack	Iced tea made in sun, Bartlett pear, small handful pecans	ROOT, FLOW, LOVE, TRUTH, INSIGHT, SPIRIT
Lunch	Grilled tuna steak on bed of arugula with sesame oil dressing, passion fruit tea, shared with a friend	ROOT, FLOW, LOVE, TRUTH, INSIGHT
Snack	Hummus with red pepper and carrots	ROOT, FLOW, FIRE
Dinner	Curried, cubed tofu with broccoli on basmati rice, cooked with gratitude	ROOT, FIRE, LOVE, INSIGHT
Snack	Mandarin	FLOW

TABLE 5. SAMPLE MENU #3

Meal	Foods	Systems
Breakfast	Homemade high-fiber, buckwheat/flax meal banana-walnut pancakes with blueberry compote	ROOT, FLOW, FIRE, LOVE, INSIGHT
Snack	Chai tea with steamed organic soy milk, warm with blessings	ROOT, LOVE, INSIGHT, SPIRIT
Lunch	Large chard leaves filled with grilled vegetables (mushroom, zucchini, red peppers, eggplant, yellow summer squash), spinach, alfalfa sprouts, avocado slices, topped with tahini	ROOT, FLOW, FIRE, LOVE, TRUTH
Snack	Eat a peach using all your senses, intentionally sip roasted green tea	FLOW, LOVE, TRUTH, INSIGHT
Dinner	Homemade turkey chili with flaxseed crackers, prayer of thanks	ROOT, FLOW, FIRE, LOVE, SPIRIT
Snack	Trail mix (mixed nuts and fruits, unsweetened, shredded coconut)	ROOT, FLOW, TRUTH

CHAPTER 13

RECIPES FOR YOUR SEVEN SYSTEMS OF HEALTH

Cooking is like love. It should be entered into with abandon or not at all.

Harriet Van Horne

These recipes are general guidelines only. Please feel free to tailor them to your specific needs as determined by your healthcare practitioner. Also, I would recommend that you choose organic food varieties whenever possible.

The ROOT System

Red Whirl Smoothie
Serves 1 to 2

2 cups frozen strawberries
1 cup frozen raspberries
1 cup unsweetened, organic milk alternative (e.g., almond, coconut)
1 tbsp. bee pollen (optional)
Handful of ice cubes
Water as needed

Combine ingredients in a blender; fill to the top with ice cubes. Add in water to make the consistency smooth.

Morning Scramble
Serves 2

3 medium-sized red potatoes, washed and cubed into 8 sections
2 tbsp. extra-virgin olive oil

2 cloves garlic, minced
1 green onion
⅛ cup black olives, sliced
1 cup broccoli florets
4 eggs
2 tbsp. unsweetened, organic milk alternative (e.g., almond, coconut)
Pinch of curry powder
Salt and pepper

Boil red potatoes in a skillet until they are slightly soft, but not mushy. Pour off any excess water from the skillet and add olive oil. Stir-fry potatoes together with garlic, green onion, olives, and broccoli florets on low heat for 2 minutes. In a small bowl, whisk together eggs, milk alternative, and curry. Pour egg mixture over stir-fry and heat, using spatula to combine ingredients periodically. Add salt and pepper to taste.

Stir-Fried Ginger-Garlic Tofu/Chicken with Vegetables
Serves 4

1 pound extra-firm organic tofu or 4 organic chicken breasts
2 tbsp. wheat-free tamari (low-sodium soy sauce)
2 tbsp. sesame oil
2 tsp. peeled and minced fresh ginger
2 minced garlic cloves
2 cups broccoli florets
2 cups sliced mushrooms
1 red bell pepper cut into thin strips
Salt and pepper to taste

Drain and cube tofu or cut up chicken breasts into bite-size pieces Toss with tamari soy sauce and 1 tbsp. oil in a small bowl and set aside for 5–10 minutes. In a wok or large non-stick skillet, heat 1 tbsp. oil over high heat and add ginger and garlic; stir-fry for 30 seconds. Add marinated tofu/chicken, stir-frying for 2 more minutes. Toss in broccoli, mushrooms, and bell pepper, and continue stir-frying for 2 minutes. Salt and pepper can be added for taste.

Earthy Chili

2 tbsp. extra-virgin olive oil
1 medium onion, chopped
4 cloves garlic, minced
½ pound mushrooms, chopped
2 cups pinto or kidney beans, cooked
1 red bell pepper, chopped
2 cups cauliflower pieces
2 carrots, scrubbed and chopped
1 28-oz. can plum tomatoes, with juice
2 tbsp. tomato paste
3 tbsp. red wine vinegar or red wine
1 cup tomato juice
1 tbsp. ground cumin
2 tbsp. chili powder
1 tsp. paprika
Salt and pepper to taste

In large soup pan, over medium heat, sauté onions and garlic in olive oil until onions become yellow and soft, about 5 minutes. Add mushrooms and sauté another 5–10 minutes. Stir in remaining ingredients and bring mixture to a boil. Reduce heat to simmer. Cover and cook, stirring occasionally, until vegetables are tender, about 50 minutes. Serve hot.

Nourishing Bean Soup

2 cups white kidney beans (cannellini)
1–2 cups kidney, adzuki, or red beans, cooked
1 cup chick peas, cooked
2–3 cups fresh spinach or escarole, washed, drained and chopped, *or*
1 10-oz. package frozen chopped spinach
4 cups organic chicken or vegetable broth
2 onions, chopped
2 cloves garlic, minced
1 tsp. each dried basil and oregano

1 tbsp. dried parsley
Pepper to taste

Combine all ingredients and simmer for 45 minutes. Serve hot.

Turkey Loaf
Serves 2 to 3

1 lb. ground free-range, organic turkey
1 egg, beaten
½ cup shiitake mushrooms, sautéed in butter
½ cup water
½ cup celery, chopped
1 small cooked red potato, diced
¼ cup organic oats
½ cup almond meal
1 tbsp. dried parsley
2 tsp. dried tarragon
1 tsp. dried sage
Sea salt and fresh ground pepper to taste

Preheat oven to 375°F. Mix all ingredients together in a bowl. Put into a casserole dish. Bake for about 35–40 minutes.

Creamy Cold Tomato Soup
Serves 3 to 4

1 cucumber, chopped
1 scallion, chopped
1 clove garlic
4 cups tomato juice, unsalted
1 red or green pepper, chopped
½ tsp. oregano
1 cup plain organic yogurt
Sliced mushrooms or tomato chunks for garnish
Salt and pepper

Combine all ingredients (except yogurt) in small amounts in blender and blend until smooth. Whisk in yogurt. Chill several hours before serving and garnish as desired with mushrooms or tomato. Add salt and pepper to taste.

Winter Root Vegetable Soup

Serves 4

2 tbsp. extra-virgin olive oil
1 ½ cups coarsely chopped onions
3 tbsp. finely chopped garlic
6 cups vegetable stock
2 tbsp. apple cider vinegar
1 pound celery root, diced (about 2 ½ cups)
¾ pound red potatoes, diced (about 2 ¾ cups)
¾ pound sweet potatoes, diced (about 2 ¾ cups)
½ pound parsnips, diced (1 ¾ cups)
½ pound carrots, diced (1 ¾ cups)
¼ pound turnips, diced (2 cups)
½ tsp. minced fresh ginger root
½ tsp. salt
¼ tsp. cumin
¼ tsp. curry
⅛ tsp. cayenne pepper

Heat the oil in a saucepan over high heat. Add the onions and sauté until soft and yellow. Add the garlic and sauté 1 minute. Add to a large soup pot along with the remaining ingredients. Simmer for 90 minutes. Serve hot.

Cinnamon-Nut Baked Apple

Serves 2

2 tbsp. cashew pieces
2 tbsp. pecan pieces
1 tbsp. unsweetened coconut flakes
1 tsp. cinnamon
2 tbsp. honey
2 apples, cored
2 tbsp. apple juice concentrate
1 cup water
2 tbsp. non-fat, plain yogurt (optional)

In a small bowl, mix together the nut pieces, unsweetened coconut flakes, cinnamon, and honey. Place cored apples in a small glass baking dish. Spoon mixture into the centers of each apple and the remainder over the tops of the apples if there is excess. Combine apple juice concentrate and water and pour over apples. Bake uncovered at 350°F for 30 minutes or until apples become soft. Serve with a dollop of non-fat yogurt as topping (optional).

The FLOW System

Honeyed Papaya with Raw Coconut Flakes   *Serves 1 to 2*

1 ripe papaya
1 tsp. honey
½ cup raw coconut flakes

Slice papaya in half, clean out seeds. Drizzle 1 tsp. honey over both halves. Sprinkle with raw coconut flakes and serve immediately.

Pleasure Fruit Mix   *Serves 2 to 3*

2 peaches, sliced
2 ripe bananas, diced
1 nectarine, sliced
1 blood orange, sectioned
1 mango, cut into thin slices
½ cup unsweetened shredded coconut
2 tbsp. lime or lemon juice
Mint sprig (optional)

Mix all ingredients except for lime/lemon juice in a large bowl. Drizzle lime or lemon juice over entire mixture. Cover and refrigerate or serve immediately. Place mint sprig on top.

Flowing Ginger Mango Smoothie   *Serves 1 to 2*

1 ripe mango, peeled and sliced
2 cups unsweetened coconut milk
2 tbsp. ground flaxseed meal
Pinch ground ginger

Blend all ingredients in blender until smooth. Serve immediately or freeze for 1 hour if you would like as a sorbet.

Grilled Salmon with Apricot-Orange
Sauce and Baby Carrots

Serves 4

24 oz. wild salmon

Sauce:

¾ cup apricot preserves
1 tbsp. teriyaki sauce
2 tbsp. balsamic vinegar
1 tsp. freshly-grated ginger
2 tbsp. sesame oil
2 tbsp. orange juice
1 tsp. orange zest
1 small bag baby carrots

Cut salmon into 4 six-ounce servings and set aside in a 9 x 13 baking pan. In small saucepan, combine apricot preserves, teriyaki sauce, vinegar, and ginger. Stir over low heat for about a minute, or until preserves become liquid. Set aside to cool to room temperature. Add sesame oil, orange juice, and orange zest and mix well. Pour ¾ of mixture on top of salmon. Cover with aluminum foil and refrigerate for 1–2 hours or until ready to grill. Keep remaining sauce on the side in a small bowl. Meanwhile, allow baby carrots to steam until they reach a soft consistency. Preheat grill to medium. Grease grill. Remove marinated salmon and place on grill. Cover grill and cook about 3–4 minutes per side or until desired doneness. Serve salmon with warm apricot sauce and baby carrots.

Creative Carrot Curry ("3 C") Soup

Serves 4

1 tbsp. extra-virgin olive oil
1 medium yellow onion, chopped finely
2 pounds carrots, scrubbed and unpeeled, cut into ½"-thick rounds
1 tbsp. curry powder
5 cups vegetable or organic chicken broth
1 cup light coconut milk
Salt and freshly ground pepper to taste

Heat the olive oil in large saucepan over medium heat. Add the chopped onion and stir 3–4 minutes or until it turns golden. Add carrots and stir well. Stir in curry powder and cook, stirring constantly, for 30 seconds. Add the broth and bring to boil over high heat. Reduce heat to medium-low and partially cover the saucepan. Simmer about 30 minutes, or until carrots are tender. In small increments, transfer soup to a blender or food processor, blending until smooth. Pour the puréed soup into large bowl. Stir in coconut milk over low heat. Season with salt and pepper and serve hot.

Wild Rice/Almond Stuffed Orange Bell Pepper   *Serves 2*

⅓ cup chopped yellow onion
1 clove garlic, minced
2 tbsp. extra-virgin olive oil
2 cups vegetable or organic chicken broth
1 cup wild rice
⅛ cup celery, diced
⅛ cup carrot, sliced into ½-inch rounds
½ cup almond slivers
⅛ tsp. rosemary
⅛ tsp. oregano
Pinch sea salt
2 large orange bell peppers, stems removed

In large saucepan, sauté onion and garlic in oil until onion becomes soft. Add broth, rice, celery, and carrot. Bring to a boil; cover, reduce heat, and simmer for 20–25 minutes or until rice is almost done. Remove from heat. Add ¼ cup almond slivers and spices. Set aside. Place peppers in large saucepan filled with 2 inches water. Bring to boil and cook for 2–3 minutes or until slightly tender. Drain water from saucepan. Place peppers in small glass casserole dish. Stuff with rice/almond mixture and spoon excess around peppers. Cover with foil and bake at 350°F for 15 minutes. Sprinkle top of peppers with almonds and serve.

Yam Pecan Bake

Serves 3 to 4

5 medium-sized yams
2 cups unsweetened coconut milk
¼ cup honey
¼ cup pecans, chopped (reserve 1 tbsp. for topping)
¼ cup unsweetened, shredded coconut (reserve 1 tbsp. for topping)
½ tsp. cinnamon
1 tsp. nutmeg

Bake yams in oven for 1 hour at 350°F or until soft. Peel off skin and put yams into large bowl. Break into small pieces using a fork. Pour coconut milk onto yams, stirring and mashing the mixture to make it smooth. Add honey, pecans, shredded coconut, cinnamon, and nutmeg and mix well. Pour into medium-sized casserole dish. Sprinkle top with reserved pecans and shredded coconut. Serve either warm or cold.

Macadamia-Encrusted Halibut

Serves 4

1 cup brown rice flour
¼ cup flaxseed meal
3 eggs
¼ cup orange juice
2 cups lightly salted roasted macadamia nuts, finely chopped
4 wild halibut fillets
¼ cup clarified butter (ghee), melted
2 tbsp. finely chopped green onion for garnish

Combine flour and flaxseed meal in a shallow bowl or plate. In a separate shallow mixing bowl, beat eggs and orange juice. Put macadamia nuts on a third shallow bowl or plate. Flour both sides of a fillet, dip in the egg bowl, and then completely cover both sides with nuts. Repeat the same procedure for all fillets. Place the fillets on a heated skillet with melted ghee and fry both sides until fish is cooked, about 10 minutes total. Sprinkle fillet with chopped green onion. Serve with mango chutney (see page 231) on side.

Fresh Almond and Cashew Nut Butter

Yields about 2 cups

1 cup unsalted roasted shelled almonds
1 cup lightly salted dry roasted cashews

Blend both nuts together in a heavy-duty blender or food processor. Store in the refrigerator in an air-tight glass jar. Use within 2 weeks.

Walnut Pesto

Yields about 3 cups

1 large head elephant garlic
1 cup extra-virgin olive oil
½ cup fresh basil leaves
1 cup walnuts (shelled)
½ cup black walnuts
1 cup pine nuts

Bake garlic in covered, oiled glass dish in oven at 350°F for about 40 minutes. Baste occasionally with olive oil. Cool and peel. Chop the basil leaves and add to blender or food processor. Add garlic, nuts, and remaining oil and mix well. Cover mixture with thin layer of oil and keep in refrigerator for up to 2 weeks.

The FIRE System

Mixed Muesli

Serves 2 to 4

1 cup unsweetened puffed rice cereal (e.g., Perky's brand)
½ cup crispy brown rice
⅛ cup oat bran
⅛ cup flaxseeds
⅛ cup unsweetened shredded coconut
¼ cup sliced almonds
⅛ cup chopped pecans
⅛ cup pumpkin seeds
¼ cup raisins
¼ cup honey
¼ cup clarified butter (ghee), melted

Mix all ingredients together in a large mixing bowl. Spread contents flat on cookie sheet. Bake at 375°F for 20 minutes or until slightly browned. Store at room temperature in a plastic or glass jar. Use as a portable snack or cereal.

Fiery Curry Lentil Soup
Serves 6

4 large garlic cloves, peeled and finely chopped
2 medium yellow onions, finely diced
1 tbsp. extra-virgin olive oil
2 cups brown and/or yellow lentils
10 cups vegetable or chicken broth
1 cup of fresh corn pieces
3–4 carrots, sliced
3 large yellow potatoes, cut into 1-inch cubes
¼ tsp. cumin
2 tsp. curry
Dash sea salt

In a small saucepan, heat garlic and onions in olive oil over medium heat until soft. Wash lentils thoroughly. In a large stock pot, add broth and all other ingredients, including the sautéed garlic and onions. Simmer and stir occasionally for at least one hour. Serve warm. Freeze unused portions.

Brown Rice with Yellow Vegetables and Sesame/Tamari Dressing
Serves 2

1 cup whole grain (short or long grain) organic brown rice (for a
    nuttier texture, choose short grain)
2 ½ cups water
2 tbsp. sesame seeds, toasted
3 tbsp. rice vinegar
2 tbsp. tamari sauce
1 tbsp. toasted sesame oil
4 tsp. minced fresh ginger
2 garlic gloves, minced or pressed
2 tsp. honey

1 cup cubed yellow squash
1 cup diced yellow bell pepper
½ cup chopped scallions

Combine rice with water in medium saucepan. Bring to a simmer over medium-high heat. Reduce heat to low and simmer, covered, until rice is tender and water has been absorbed, 30–35 minutes. Fluff with fork and transfer to large bowl. Alternately, cook rice in rice cooker. While rice is cooking, toast sesame seeds in small dry skillet over medium-low heat, stirring constantly until golden and fragrant, about 3 minutes. Cool in small bowl. Whisk together vinegar, tamari sauce, oil, ginger, garlic and honey in another small bowl. Add this mixture to rice when cooled and toss to coat well. Add yellow squash, yellow bell pepper, and scallions, and toss to coat. Sprinkle with sesame seeds before serving.

Quinoa/Amaranth Pine Nut Salad

Serves 2

1 cup quinoa, rinsed
1 cup amaranth, rinsed
3 cups water
Pinch sea salt
½ cup corn kernels
½ medium cucumber, diced
1 medium tomato, diced
½ cup chopped cilantro
½ cup chopped basil
2 tbsp. lemon juice
1 cup pine nuts
Pepper

Combine quinoa, amaranth, water, and salt in a medium-sized covered saucepan. Bring to boil, simmer 20 minutes. In medium-sized glass bowl, mix together corn, cucumber, tomato, cilantro, basil, and lemon juice. Add to quinoa mixture. Mix well. Toss in pine nuts before serving. Sprinkle with pepper to taste. Serve warm or cold.

Mediterranean Polenta Medallions   *Serves 2*

1 roll precooked compressed polenta, sliced
2 tbsp. extra-virgin olive oil
½ cup basil, chopped
1 tsp. oregano
1 medium tomato, diced
½ cup pine nuts
¼ cup feta cheese
Dash sea salt
Dash pepper

Arrange polenta slices on an oiled skillet and heat over medium heat, flip-
ping over after about 1 minute, until polenta turns slightly brown. Empty
toasted polenta onto large plate. On top of polenta, add basil, oregano,
tomato, pine nuts, and feta cheese. Salt and pepper to taste.

Sunny Corn Salad   *Serves 2 to 4*

6–8 ears fresh corn or 3 cups frozen corn kernels
1 large red bell pepper, diced
3 green onions, cut into ¼-inch pieces
⅛ cup extra-virgin olive oil
2 tbsp. lemon juice
1–2 cloves garlic, minced
¼ cup cilantro
⅛ tsp. chili powder
1–2 jalapenos, diced
Salt and pepper to taste

Combine all ingredients in a medium-sized glass mixing bowl. Serve cold.

Brown Rice Pudding   *Serves 4*

2 cups brown rice
4 cups water
½ cup unsweetened coconut milk
1 tsp. cinnamon
½ tsp. cardamom

1 scant handful pecan pieces
¼ cup honey

Rinse rice well. Add to medium saucepan with water. Cover and cook 20–25 minutes or until rice is done. Stir in coconut milk, cinnamon, cardamom, and pecan pieces. Stir in honey. Serve warm or cold.

The LOVE System

Flax/Zucchini Muffins of Joy   *Yields about 6 muffins*

1 ½ cups brown rice flour
1 cup flaxseed meal
2 tsp. baking soda
1 tsp. baking powder
½ tsp. sea salt
2 tsp. cinnamon
½ tsp. cardamom
½ cup raisins
1 cup pecans, chopped
1 ½ cups zucchini, shredded
1 cup honey
¾ cup unsweetened alternative milk (e.g., almond, coconut)
2 eggs, beaten
1 tsp. vanilla

In a large bowl, mix together dry ingredients (flour, flaxseed meal, baking soda, baking powder, sea salt, cinnamon, cardamom, raisins, pecans). In a separate bowl, combine zucchini, honey, milk alternative, beaten eggs, and vanilla. Pour combined liquid ingredients into dry-ingredient mixture. Stir by hand until ingredients are moistened. Grease medium-sized muffin pan with organic coconut oil. Fill each muffin well about ¾ full with batter. Bake at 375°F for 15–20 minutes or until slightly browned. Allow to cool before eating. Stores well in freezer.

The Heart Salad
Serves 3 to 4

1 bag fresh organic spinach leaves (10–12 oz.)
1 ripe avocado, diced into cubes
1 cup broccoli sprouts
1 tsp. fresh dill
½ cup strawberries, sliced in half (to resemble heart shape)
½ cup toasted slivered almonds
Dash sea salt and pepper

Dressing:
¼ cup flaxseed oil
¼ cup extra-virgin olive oil
¼ cup balsamic vinegar

Wash spinach leaves and put into large serving bowl. Add avocado cubes, broccoli sprouts, and dill, and lightly mix throughout. Top with strawberries and almonds. Combine dressing ingredients in shaker cup. Before serving, drizzle salad with dressing. Add salt and pepper to taste.

Rosemary Roasted Cauliflower and Pine Nuts
Serves 2 to 3

1 large head organic cauliflower
2 cloves of garlic, peeled and minced
⅛ cup extra-virgin olive oil
1 tbsp. fresh rosemary
½ cup raw pine nuts
Sea salt
Fresh-ground pepper

Preheat oven to 425°F. Break apart cauliflower into bite-sized pieces or florets and place in large mixing bowl. Add garlic and stir throughout. Pour in olive oil and ensure that all cauliflower pieces are drizzled with oil. Sprinkle with rosemary, pine nuts, salt and pepper. Transfer mixture evenly onto baking sheet and set, uncovered, in oven for 20–25 minutes or until the top and edges of cauliflower are lightly brown. Serve immediately.

Heart-Warming Brussels Sprouts   *Serves 2 to 3*

1 lb. fresh Brussels sprouts, washed and cut in half
1 small yellow onion, peeled and chopped
2 tbsp. clarified butter (ghee)
Dash sea salt and pepper
2 tbsp. freshly grated Parmesan cheese (optional)

Steam Brussels sprouts for 2–3 minutes or until bright green and tender. Sauté onions in 1 tbsp. ghee until they become translucent. Add steamed Brussels sprouts and the remaining ghee. Toss, sprinkle with salt and pepper to taste, and cook on medium high heat until Brussels sprouts turn slightly brown. Remove from heat, put into serving dish. Sprinkle top with grated Parmesan cheese.

Thank You Rice Paper Rolls   *Makes 4 to 6 rolls*

1 package of rice paper wrappers
Several leaves of romaine or iceberg lettuce
1 cup white jasmine rice, cooked and cooled
1 cup cilantro, washed and chopped
¼ cup cucumber, washed and cut into small cubes
⅛ cup carrots, shredded
1 cup bean sprouts
1 cup extra-firm organic tofu, cubed
or
1 cup of baby pre-cooked shrimp, rinsed well
1 tbsp. crushed peanuts

Pour hot water into a shallow wide bowl that will fit the diameter of the rice paper wrapper. Gently take a rice paper wrapper from the package and place it into the bowl of warm water. Allow it to sit for a minute or until it becomes soft. Once soft, remove and place on a clean cutting board or large plate. Put lettuce leaf on top, and then add small amounts of rice, cilantro, cucumber, carrots, bean sprouts, tofu/shrimp, and crushed peanuts. Roll up the wrap tightly and tuck in edges. Serve rolls plain or with a dipping sauce (see page 230).

Heart-y Split Pea Soup

Serves 3 to 4

1 tbsp. extra-virgin olive oil
1 small yellow onion, diced
1 bay leaf
3 cloves garlic, peeled and minced
2 cups dried green split peas
1 ½ tsp. sea salt
11 cups water
2 carrots, chopped
1 leek, chopped
3 celery stalks, chopped
½ cup parsley, chopped
½ tsp. dried basil
Dash fresh ground pepper

In a large pot over medium high heat, sauté oil, onion, bay leaf, and garlic for 3–4 minutes or until onions are soft and translucent. Add the peas, salt, and water. Bring to boil and reduce heat to low. Simmer for 90 minutes, stirring occasionally. Add the carrots, leek, celery, parsley, basil, and ground pepper. Simmer for about 45 minutes, or until peas and vegetables are tender.

Green Garbanzo Beans with Love Rice

Serves 4

1 cup dried green garbanzo beans
1 ½ cups brown basmati rice
½ tsp. sea salt
½ cup walnuts
1 handful basil
2 cloves garlic
1 tbsp. lemon juice
2 tbsp. extra-virgin olive oil
½ cup celery, diced
Fresh ground pepper to taste

Bring water to boil and add beans, rice, and salt. Simmer, covered, for about 40 minutes. Remove from heat and let sit with cover on for about

10 minutes. Remove cover and allow to cool. While beans and rice are cooking, blend walnuts, basil, garlic, lemon juice, and olive oil in a food processor. When beans and rice are cool, stir in nut-basil mixture and celery. Add pepper to taste.

Sesame Kale and Spinach Tango

Serves 2 to 3

1 bag fresh organic spinach, washed
1 bunch dinosaur kale, washed, chopped
1 green onion, chopped
2 cloves garlic, peeled and minced
1 tsp. sesame seeds
1 tbsp. sesame oil

In a covered saucepan, cook spinach and kale on medium heat until wilted, but still bright green. While greens are cooking, use separate pan to stir-fry green onion, garlic, and sesame seeds in sesame oil until sesame seeds are slightly browned. Add to drained, cooked greens, mix well and serve either hot or chilled.

The TRUTH System

Spicy Nut Sauce

Yields about 1 cup

½ cup organic crunchy peanut butter
½ cup organic cashew nut butter
4 tbsp. black or green tea
1 tsp. sesame oil
2 tbsp. wheat-free tamari sauce
1 tbsp. rice vinegar
1 tsp. honey
1 clove garlic, peeled and minced
¼ tsp. crushed red pepper

Combine all ingredients. Spoon over steamed green vegetables or use as dipping sauce for rice or vegetable rolls.

Mango Chutney

Makes about 2 to 3 cups

1 tbsp. sesame oil
1 tsp. cayenne pepper
1 tbsp. curry powder
¾ cup diced yellow onion
2 tbsp. minced fresh ginger
½ cup golden raisins
½ cup diced orange bell pepper
3 cups fresh, ripe mangoes (roughly 2 mangoes), peeled and cut
   into strips
½ cup unsweetened pineapple juice
½ cup apple cider vinegar
1 cup honey

In a small skillet, heat the oil and add the cayenne pepper, curry powder, and onions. Once onions become soft, add the ginger, raisins, and bell pepper and continue sautéing for 1 minute. Add the mango and cook for another minute. In a small mixing bowl, combine the pineapple juice, vinegar, and honey. Add this mixture to the skillet. Simmer on low heat, stirring frequently, for 20–25 minutes, or until slightly thickened. Allow to cool, and pour into glass jar for storage.

Balsamic Vinegar/Peach Sauce

Makes about 1 cup

½ cup balsamic vinegar
½ cup peaches, chopped
2 tbsp. dried cranberries
1 tbsp. walnut oil
1 tbsp. walnuts, chopped

Simmer balsamic vinegar with peaches in a small skillet over medium heat until it turns to a syrup-like texture (about 1 ½ minutes). Remove from heat. Add dried cranberries, walnut oil, and walnuts. Drizzle on vegetables or chill and use as a salad dressing.

Sea Plant Veggies

Serves 2

1 cup dulse, soaked and sliced into bite-sized bits
1 cup shredded carrots
1 cup alfalfa sprouts
3 red radishes, sliced
1 tsp. sesame oil
1 tbsp. sesame seeds
Pinch sea salt

In mixing bowl, combine all ingredients. Serve cold.

Vegetable Nori Rolls

Makes 6 rolls

2 cups cooked brown rice
2 tbsp. rice vinegar
6 sheets pressed nori

Filling:

¼ cup grated cucumber
¼ cup alfalfa sprouts
¼ cup purple cabbage
1 tsp. wheat-free tamari or soy sauce
1 tsp. sesame seeds

Combine all ingredients for filling and set aside. Mix vinegar into rice. Place a single sheet of nori on a heavy cloth napkin to facilitate rolling. Spread ½ cup rice over the sheet, leaving about a 1–2-inch edge. Put ¼ cup of filling down the middle on the flattened rice. Roll the nori. Eat as long nori stick, or cut to 1-inch pieces.

Asian Miso-Dulse Soup

Serves 2 to 3

5 cups water
1 ½ cups shredded bok choy and Chinese cabbage
3 large shiitake mushrooms, sliced
1 green onion, finely chopped
1 cup dulse
3 tbsp. red miso

1 cup of extra-firm organic tofu, cubed *or*
1 cup organic chicken, cubed
Sea salt, pinch

In a pot, add water, bok choy, cabbage, mushrooms, onion, dulse, and miso, and heat on low-to-medium heat for about 10 minutes. Add the tofu or chicken, and salt, if needed. Serve immediately.

Sea Slaw

Serves 2 to 3

1 small red cabbage, grated or chopped
1 small green cabbage, grated or chopped
2 carrots, grated
1 cup dulse, soaked and sliced
2 tbsp. orange juice
½ cup apple cider vinegar
1 tbsp. caraway seeds
Sea salt and fresh ground pepper to taste

Combine ingredients and serve cold.

The INSIGHT System

Green Tea/Berry Freeze

Serves 2

1 cup water
2 green tea bags
2 cups frozen mixed berries (blueberries, raspberries, blackberries)
1 ½ cups organic coconut milk
¼ cup pomegranate juice

Boil water and add to tea bags. Steep for 5 minutes. In meantime, combine mixed berries, milk, and juice in a blender until smooth. Add tea to berry blend. Drink as a smoothie or freeze if you prefer to eat as a sorbet.

Choco-ffee Tofu INSIGHT Whip
Serves 2 to 3

1 10-oz. package of firm, organic tofu, drained
½ cup honey
¼ tsp. cinnamon
¼ tsp. cardamom
1 tsp. instant coffee
1 tsp. shredded unsweetened coconut
2 tbsp. cocoa
½ tsp. vanilla

Blend all ingredients until smooth. Place in a bowl, cover, and chill for 3–4 hours.

Ch-Eye Tea
Serves 2 to 3

4 tsp. loose black (e.g., Darjeeling) or green tea
1 cup water
¼-inch ginger root, sliced thin
1 cinnamon stick, crushed
6 cardamom pods, crushed
3 cloves
2 cups milk alternative of your choice (coconut is a good choice for this one!)
Honey to taste, optional

In a saucepan, boil tea in 1 cup water. Allow to steep for 5 minutes. Add ginger, cinnamon, cardamom, cloves, and milk alternative. Heat mixture on low to medium-high heat for 2 minutes, stirring occasionally. Remove from heat. Let sit for 2 minutes. Add honey to sweeten. Serve warm.

Berry Wisdom-Seeker Cobbler
Serves 2 to 3

2 cups blueberries
1 cup blackberries
¼ cup honey
¼ tsp. cinnamon
¼ tsp. vanilla extract
1 cup organic rolled oats (not instant)

¼ tsp. stevia

3 tbsp. brown rice flour, sifted

1 ½ tbsp. organic butter, softened

Preheat oven to 350°F. Gently mix both berries, honey, cinnamon, and vanilla in a medium-sized bowl. Place in an 8-inch baking pan. In separate bowl, combine oats, stevia, brown rice flour, and butter. Mix with fingers until all ingredients are crumbly. Spoon on top of fruit mixture. Bake 35–40 minutes or until slightly browned. Cool before serving. Serve with organic vanilla yogurt.

Ginger Spice Bread
Serves 4 to 6

2 cups brown rice flour

1 ½ tsp. baking soda

2 tsp. ground ginger

1 tsp. cardamom

1 tsp. cinnamon

1 tsp. nutmeg

½ tsp. sea salt

2 eggs

½ cup honey

½ cup unsulphured molasses

2 tbsp. fresh grated ginger

½ cup apple juice

¼ cup organic canola oil

1 tsp. orange zest

Preheat oven to 350°F. In a medium bowl, combine all dry ingredients: flour, baking soda, ground ginger, cardamom, cinnamon, nutmeg, sea salt. In a separate, large bowl, mix together eggs, honey, molasses, fresh ginger, apple juice, oil, and orange zest. Slowly blend the dry mixture into the liquid ingredients so that they are evenly mixed. Pour into an 8-inch square baking pan. Bake for 30 minutes or until slightly browned. Cool before cutting and removing from pan. Cut into squares and serve.

The SPIRIT System

Detox Dynamo

Serves 1

Intention of "clarity"
1 organic apple (red or green), cored
1 organic carrot
1 organic celery stalk
½-inch ginger root
½ whole lemon
1 handful organic spinach leaves
Pinch cayenne pepper
Water as needed

With intention, juice all fruits and vegetables in a juicer. Add cayenne pepper, stir, and drink mindfully.

Berry Flush

Serves 1

1 organic Red Delicious or Pink Lady apple, cored
1 cup organic strawberries, sliced
1 cup organic blueberries
½ cup organic blackberries
Pinch cinnamon
Water as needed

Blend all ingredients in a blender or juicer. Infuse final mixture with "love" and "universal light and peace." Sip intentionally.

Sun-and-Fruit Water

1 gallon purified water
Sunny day
½ organic cucumber, sliced
2 slices organic orange
3 strawberries, sliced thinly, tops removed

Put water in a large glass pitcher in sunlight for 3–6 hours (10 a.m. to 4 p.m.). Add fruit. Gently stir. Sip throughout day.

Green Goddess

Serves 1

1 organic cucumber
1 cup organic broccoli sprouts
1 stalk organic celery
1 organic green apple, cored
⅛ cup chopped mint
1 handful (organic) barley grass

Juice all ingredients in a juicer. Drink with intention.

Divine Broth

Serves 1 to 2

5 cups purified water
1 organic carrot, sliced
1 stalk organic celery, diced
½ cup parsley, chopped
1 organic green onion, finely sliced
½ cup chopped organic leeks
¼ cup burdock root, chopped
1 tbsp. fresh squeezed lemon juice
Sprinkle coarse sea salt

Boil water and add all ingredients. Gently simmer for 30 minutes. Serve warm.

ACKNOWLEDGMENTS

I am incredibly grateful to all involved for the opportunity to share this creation, which is really an aggregation of the inspiration, insight, and information received from numerous teachers, mentors, and friends who have formed ripples in my internal waters throughout my life.

Heartfelt thanks also go to my family for their bountiful gifts: my mother for her strength and faith; my father for his ability to love unconditionally; my sister for her keen wit and creativity; and my brother for his depth and understanding. My partner, Mark, has been supportive of the time and space I have needed to write. He continues to teach me the power of the middle path. My agent, Krista Goering, has been wonderfully patient with the process and helpful in getting this work out to the world.

Truly, I am in awe of all the people I have met on my life path who have sought wisdom and healing in classes I've offered or during clinic visits. Thank you for allowing me into your lives to give and receive what I could. I remain in service to you.

APPENDIX A

THE SEVEN SYSTEMS OF FULL-SPECTRUM HEALTH

THE SEVEN SYSTEMS OF FULL-SPECTRUM HEALTH

System	Endocrine Gland	Anatomy	Physiological Activities	Core Issues	Food
▢ The Root	Adrenal Glands	• Adrenal glands • Blood cells • Bones • DNA • Feet • Immune System • Joints • Legs • Muscles • Rectum • Skin • Tailbone (Coccyx)	• Enzyme activity • Fight-or-flight response • Gene expression • Protein production	• Safety • Survival • Tribe	• Dietary proteins • Immune-enhancing foods • Insoluble fiber • Mineral-rich foods • Red-colored foods • Root vegetables
◯ The Flow	Ovaries/ testes	• Bladder • Hips • Kidneys • Large intestine • Ovaries • Reproductive system • Sacrum • Testes	• Cellular replication • Fat storage • Reproduction • Water balance	• Creativity • Emotions • Relationships	• Dietary fats and oils • Fermented foods • Fish and seafood • Nuts and seeds • Orange-colored foods • Tropical foods • Water

System	Endocrine Gland	Anatomy	Physiological Activities	Core Issues	Food
△ The Fire	Pancreas	• Gallbladder • Liver • Pancreas • Small intestine • Stomach	• Assimilation • Biotransformation • Blood sugar balance • Digestion	• Balance • Energy • Power	• Dietary carbohydrates • Healthy sweeteners • Legumes • Soluble fiber • Whole grains • Yellow-colored foods
◇ The Love	Thymus and Heart	• Armpits • Arms • Blood vessels • Breasts • Hands • Heart • Lungs • Lymphatic system • Shoulders • Thymus • Wrists	• Breathing • Circulation • Oxygenation	• Compassion • Expansion • Service	• Leafy vegetables • Microgreens • Phytonutrients • Sprouts • Vegetables (especially green)
☆ The Truth	Thyroid Gland	• Cheeks • Chin • Ears • Mouth • Neck • Nose • Throat • Thyroid gland	• Chewing • Metabolism • Hearing • Smelling • Speaking	• Authenticity • Choice • Voice	• Fruits • Juice • Sauces • Sea plants • Soups • Teas
◎ The Insight	Pituitary Gland	• Brain • Eyebrows • Eyes • Forehead • Neurons • Neurotransmitters • Pituitary gland	• Mood balance • Sleep • Thought processing	• Intuition • Reflection • Visualization	• Blue-purple foods • Caffeine • Chocolate/cocoa • Mood-modulating foods • Spices
✷ The Spirit	Pineal gland	• Electromagnetic field • Energy meridians • Nervous system • Pineal gland	• Circadian rhythms • Cleansing • Light sensitivity and receptivity	• Connection • Purpose • Soul	• Fasting and detoxification practices • No foods • Photons • Toxin-free foods

REFERENCE GUIDE TO HEALTH CONDITIONS FOR THE SEVEN SYSTEMS OF HEALTH

Key ❖ Primary system affected
√ Secondary system(s) affected

	ROOT	FLOW	FIRE	LOVE	TRUTH	INSIGHT	SPIRIT
Adrenal gland dysfunction	❖						
Aging/Oxidative stress	√	√	√				❖
Allergic rhinitis	√				❖		
Altered taste perception					❖		
Anemia	❖						
Blood lipid abnormalities				❖			
Blood sugar imbalance			❖				
Bone disorders	❖						
Breast health				❖			
Circulation disorders	√			❖			
Common cold	❖				√		
Depression	√					❖	√
Digestive tract dysfunction		√	❖				
Fatigue/low energy production	√		❖				√

	ROOT	FLOW	FIRE	LOVE	TRUTH	INSIGHT	SPIRIT
Hearing loss					❖		
Hormonal conditions		❖					
Immune disorders	❖				√		
Infections	❖				√		
Inflammatory conditions	❖		√				
Insomnia						❖	
Liver dysfunction			❖				
Low stomach-acid production (achlorhydria)	√		❖				
Memory loss						❖	
Nervous system disorders			√				❖
Prostate health	❖						
Protein maldigestion	√		❖				
Sore throat					❖		
Stomach upset			❖				
Thyroid dysfunction					❖		
Urinary tract conditions		❖					
Wound healing	❖						

HERBS AND SUPPLEMENTS FOR THE SEVEN SYSTEMS OF HEALTH

Key ✧ Primary system
● Secondary system(s)

	ROOT	FLOW	FIRE	LOVE	TRUTH	INSIGHT	SPIRIT
Vitamins							
Multivitamin							✧
Vitamin A	✧	●	●	●	●	●	
Vitamin B Complex			✧				
Vitamin B1 (Benfotiamine, fat soluble)			●				✧
Vitamin B1 (Thiamin, water soluble)			✧				●
Vitamin B2 (Riboflavin)	●		✧				
Vitamin B3 (Niacin)			✧	●			
Vitamin B5 (Pantothenic acid)	●		✧				
Vitamin B6 (Pyridoxine)	●	●	✧	●		●	●
Vitamin B7 (Biotin)	●		✧				●

	ROOT	FLOW	FIRE	LOVE	TRUTH	INSIGHT	SPIRIT
Vitamin B9 (Folic acid)	☼	●		●		●	
Vitamin B12 (Cyanocobalamin)	☼		●	●		●	●
Vitamin C (Ascorbic acid)	☼				●	●	●
Vitamin D (Cholecalciferol)	☼				●	●	●
Vitamin E (Tocopherols)		☼		●		●	●
Vitamin K (Phylloquinone)	●			☼			
Minerals							
Calcium	☼	●		●		●	●
Chromium			☼				
Copper	☼						
Iodine				●	☼		
Iron	☼						
Magnesium	●	●	●	☼	●	●	●
Phosphorus	☼	●	●			●	
Potassium				☼		●	●
Selenium	●	☼	●		●		
Zinc	☼				●		
Other							
5-hydroxytryptophan						☼	
Acetyl-L-carnitine						☼	
Aloe vera		☼					
Alpha lipoic acid			☼				●
Amino acids (protein)	☼					●	
Andrographis	☼		●		●		
Ashwagandha	☼		●				

	ROOT	FLOW	FIRE	LOVE	TRUTH	INSIGHT	SPIRIT
Astragalus	✿		●		●		
Bearberry leaf		✿					
Beta-carotene		✿					
Betaine hydrochloride	●		✿				
Bilberry fruit extract				✿		●	
Bioflavonoids				✿			
Bitter melon			✿				
Black cohosh		✿					
Blue-green algae					✿		
Brahmi						✿	
Bromelain	●		✿	●			
Brown seaweed					✿		
Butterbur						✿	
Cat's claw	✿						
Chasteberry fruit		✿					
Choline			✿			●	●
Chondroitin sulfate	✿						
Cinnamon			✿				
Coenzyme Q10				✿			●
Cordyceps	✿		●				
Cranberry extract	●	✿					
Curcumin	●		✿				
Dandelion root			✿				
Dang Shen	✿		●				
Digestive enzymes			✿				
Docosahexaenoic acid (DHA)		✿				●	●

	ROOT	FLOW	FIRE	LOVE	TRUTH	INSIGHT	SPIRIT
Echinacea	✿				●		
Eicosapentaenoic acid (EPA)		✿				●	●
Elderberry	✿				●		
Eleuthero	✿		●				
Fenugreek			✿				
Fish oils	●	✿		●		●	●
Five-flavor berry	✿		●				
Garlic				✿			
Ginger root			✿				
Ginseng, American			✿				
Ginseng, Panax	✿		●				
Glucosamine sulfate	✿				●		
Gotu kola				✿		●	●
Grapeseed extract				✿		●	
Green food powders				✿			
Green tea extract			✿			●	
Gymnema			✿				
Hawthorn				✿			
Hesperidin				✿			
Holy basil	✿		●				
Hops						✿	
Horse chestnut				✿			
Indian Frankincense	✿						
Indole-3-carbinol/DIM				✿			
Inositol (myo-inositol)		●				✿	●

	ROOT	FLOW	FIRE	LOVE	TRUTH	INSIGHT	SPIRIT
L-arginine	●			✿			
L-carnitine			✿				
Lemon balm						✿	
Licorice	✿		●		●		
L-theanine						✿	
Lutein						✿	
Lycopene	✿			●			
Marshmallow					✿		
Melatonin						✿	
Methylsulfonyl-methane (MSM)	✿				●		
Milk thistle			✿				
Passionflower						✿	
Phosphati-dylserine						✿	
Phytosterols	●			✿			
Plant oils		✿				●	●
Prebiotics	●	✿	●				
Probiotics	●	✿			●		
Quercetin				✿			
Red clover		✿					
Red yeast rice				✿			
Reishi	✿		●				
Resveratrol							✿
Rhodiola rosea	✿		●				
Rutin				✿			
Saw palmetto	✿						
Slippery elm					✿		
Soy isoflavones		✿					
Soy protein	●			✿			
St. John's wort						✿	

	ROOT	FLOW	FIRE	LOVE	TRUTH	INSIGHT	SPIRIT
Stinging nettle					✿		
Turmeric	●		✿				
Valerian root						✿	
Willow bark	✿						
Zeaxanthin						✿	

APPENDIX D

SPECTRUM QUIZ SCORE TRACKER

Use this table to track your scores for each system of health over time, according to your Spectrum Quiz results. Remember that a score greater than 15 is considered an imbalance.

SPECTRUM QUIZ SCORES FOR THE SEVEN SYSTEMS OF HEALTH

Date	ROOT	FLOW	FIRE	LOVE	TRUTH	INSIGHT	SPIRIT

RESOURCES

Whole Detox Programs

To find out about participating in Dr. Minich's colorful Whole Detox programs, visit these websites:

> Food & Spirit at *www.drdeannaminich.com*
> Whole Detox at *www.whole-detox.com*

The Whole Detox program is a twenty-one-day program that is available online throughout the year. The online experience gives you the opportunity to follow the program as outlined in the Whole Detox book, with the support of a larger community accessed through a private social media (Facebook) group page.

Practitioners

If you want to work with a Certified Food & Spirit Practitioner who has been trained in the seven systems of health, you can find a web directory, along with information about becoming a Certified Food & Spirit Practitioner at

> *www.foodandspirit.com*

Learn more about functional medicine and find a Certified Functional Medicine Practitioner at

> *www.functionalmedicine.org*

Social Media

Deanna Minich, PhD:

- *www.facebook.com/deanna.minich*
- *https://twitter.com/drdeannaminich*
- *https://youtube.com/channel/UCehMfF-PkIOfNsZ1Ed9WvMA*
- *https://pinterest.com/foodandspirit*
- *https://www.instagram.com/deannaminich/*

Other Books and Materials by Dr. Deanna Minich

These are resources that can support you on your path to greater health and wellness. They are all available at *www.amazon.com*.

- *An A-Z Guide to Food Additives: Never Eat What You Can't Pronounce* (Conari Press, 2009). A small pocketbook listing the important additives in foods. What's good and what's not? This book rates ingredients and foods using a simple scoring system of A through F. It is concise and targeted for the busy consumer. Make sure you have this in your purse, handbag, or pocket while shopping!

- *The Complete Handbook of Quantum Healing: An A-Z Self-Healing Guide for Over 100 Common Ailments* (Conari Press, 2010). This reference book is full of nutrition and lifestyle suggestions for specific ailments. You may want to review it for specific ailments that you have so you can fine tune your detox modalities to fit your specific needs.

- *Nourish Your Whole Self 56-Card Deck* (Self-published, 2013). The fifty-six cards in this creative, inspirational deck each carry an affirmation and visual to add greater nourishment to your eating experience. Pick a card before, during, or after a meal—or even at the start of the day—to see what eating message is waiting for you. Read more about the card you chose in the accompanying card booklet.

- *Whole Detox: A 21-Day Personalized Program to Break Through Barriers in Every Area of Your Life* (HarperOne, 2016). This book provides a step-by-step program for using the seven systems of health to remove any toxins or barriers to your health.

Recommended Products

Seafood

- Get quality fish and seafood at Vital Choice (*www.vitalchoice.com*)

Teas

- Teeccino gluten-free herbal teas (*www.teeccino.com*).
- Rishi Teas (*www.rishi-tea.com*)
- Pukka Herbs (*www.pukkaherbs.com*)
- Yogi Teas (*www.yogiproducts.com*)

Seaweeds

- Make sure your edible seaweeds are organically certified and carefully harvested. Maine Coast Sea Vegetables specializes in sustainably harvested seaweeds from the North Atlantic (*www.seaveg.com/shop*).

Spices

- Teeny Tiny Spice Co. of Vermont has a wide variety of mixed spices (e.g., tandoori masala, vindaloo, etc.) (*www.teenytinyspice.com*).
- Single spices or simple blends are available at Simply Organic (*www.simplyorganic.com*). Frontier Natural Product brands are also a good source. (*www.iherb.com/frontier-natural-products*)

Green Food Powders

- Whole-food, green food powders are available from pHresh Greens (*www.phreshproducts.com*).

Supplements

High-quality, reliable supplements are available from the following sources:

- Allergy Research Group (*www.allergyresearchgroup.com*)
- Biotics Research (*www.bioticsresearch.com*)
- Designs for Health (*www.designsforhealth.com*)
- Douglas Laboratories (*www.douglaslabs.com*)
- Innate Response (*www.innateresponse.com*)
- Metagenics, Inc. (*www.metagenics.com*)
- ProThera/Klaire Labs (*www.protherainc.com*)
- Pure Encapsulations (*www.pureencapsulations.com*)
- Thorne Research (*www.thorne.com*)
- Vital Nutrients (*www.vitalnutrients.net*)
- Xymogen (*www.xymogen.com*)

Informational Websites

These websites provide you with information on lifestyle medicine, nutrition, and personal growth that may be useful to you:

- American College of Nutrition (*www.americancollegeofnutrition.org*)
- Blogs, videos, and information on mind and body (*www.mindbodygreen.com*)
- Environmental Working Group (*www.ewg.org*)
- Find a yoga teacher at Yoga Alliance (*www.yogaalliance.org*)
- HeartMath for biofeedback and heart rate variability devices (*www.heartmath.com* and *www.heartmath.org*)
- Information on personalized lifestyle medicine from Dr. Jeffrey Bland (*www.plminstitute.org*)
- Information on toxic substances and health (*www.greenmedinfo.com*)
- Practical information on nutrition (*http://whfoods.com*)

BIBLIOGRAPHY

References are listed in order of mention within each chapter.

General References

Balch JF and Balch PA. *Prescription for Nutritional Healing.* New York: Avery Publishing Group, 1990.

Jellin JM, ed. *Natural Medicines Comprehensive Database.* Available at *www. naturaldatabase.com.*

U.S. National Library of Medicine and National Institutes of Health, PUBMED. Available at *www.ncbi.nlm.nih.gov/pubmed.*

Stargrove MB, Treasure J, McKee DL. *Herb, Nutrient, and Drug Interactions.* St. Louis, MO: Elsevier, 2008.

Chapter 3. Eating for Your Inner Rainbow

Sebeková K, Somoza V. Dietary advanced glycation endproducts (AGEs) and their health effects—PRO. *Mol Nutr Food Res.* 2007 Sep;51(9):1079-84.

Hogervorst JG, Baars BJ, Schouten LJ, Konings EJ, Goldbohm RA, van den Brandt PA. The carcinogenicity of dietary acrylamide intake: a comparative discussion of epidemiological and experimental animal research. *Crit Rev Toxicol.* 2010 Jul;40(6):485–512. doi: 10.3109/10408440903524254.

Chapter 4. Supplements

Council for Responsible Nutrition. Dietary Supplements: Safe, Beneficial and Regulated. Available at *www.crnusa.org.*

Chapter 5. The Red ROOT

Reddy P, Edwards LR. Magnesium Supplementation in Vitamin D Deficiency. *Am J Ther.* 2017 May 3.

Sluijs I, Beulens JW, van der A DL, Spijkerman AM, Grobbee DE, van der Schouw YT. Dietary intake of total, animal, and vegetable protein and risk of type-2 diabetes in the European Prospective Investigation into Cancer and Nutrition (EPIC)-NL study. *Diabetes Care.* 2010 Jan;33(1):43–8. doi: 10.2337/dc09–1321. Epub 2009 Oct 13.

Sellmeyer DE, Stone KL, Sebastian A, Cummings SR. A high ratio of dietary animal to vegetable protein increases the rate of bone loss and the risk of fracture in postmenopausal women. Study of Osteoporotic Fractures Research Group. *Am J Clin Nutr.* 2001 Jan;73(1):118–22.

Pedersen AN, Kondrup J, Børsheim E. Health effects of protein intake in healthy adults: a systematic literature review. *Food Nutr Res.* 2013 Jul 30;57. doi: 10.3402/fnr.v57i0.21245. Print 2013.

Rebholz CM, Friedman EE, Powers LJ, Arroyave WD, He J, Kelly TN. Dietary protein intake and blood pressure: a meta-analysis of randomized controlled trials. *Am J Epidemiol.* 2012 Oct 1;176 Suppl 7:S27–43. doi: 10.1093/aje/kws245.

Jesudason D, Clifton P. The interaction between dietary protein and bone health. *J Bone Miner Metab.* 2011 Jan;29(1):1–14. doi: 10.1007/s00774–010-0225-9. Epub 2010 Oct 26.

Massey LK. Dietary animal and plant protein and human bone health: a whole foods approach. *J Nutr.* 2003 Mar;133(3):862S–865S.

Scialla JJ, Anderson CA. Dietary acid load: a novel nutritional target in chronic kidney disease? *Adv Chronic Kidney Dis.* 2013 Mar;20(2):141–9. doi: 10.1053/j.ackd.2012.11.001.

Welch AA, Mulligan A, Bingham SA, Khaw KT. Urine pH is an indicator of dietary acid-base load, fruit and vegetables and meat intakes: results from the European Prospective Investigation into Cancer and Nutrition (EPIC)—Norfolk population study. *Br J Nutr.* 2008 Jun;99(6):1335–43. Epub 2007 Nov 28.

Welch AA, Bingham SA, Reeve J, Khaw KT. More acidic dietary acid-base load is associated with reduced calcaneal broadband ultrasound attenuation in women but not in men: results from the EPIC—Norfolk cohort study. *Am J Clin Nutr.* 2007 Apr;85(4):1134–41.

Barański M, Srednicka-Tober D, Volakakis N, Seal C, Sanderson R, Stewart GB, Benbrook C, Biavati B, Markellou E, Giotis C, Gromadzka-Ostrowska J, Rembiałkowska E, Skwarło-Sońta K, Tahvonen R, Janovská D, Niggli U, Nicot P, Leifert C. Higher antioxidant and lower cadmium concentrations and lower incidence of pesticide residues in organically grown crops: a systematic literature review and meta-analyses. *Br J Nutr.* 2014 Sep 14;112(5):794-811. doi: 10.1017/S0007114514001366. Epub 2014 Jun 26.

Hussain A, Larsson H, Kuktaite R, Johansson E. Mineral composition of organically grown wheat genotypes: contribution to daily minerals intake. *Int J Environ Res Public Health.* 2010 Sep;7(9):3442–56. doi: 10.3390/ijerph7093442. Epub 2010 Sep 6.

Singh AK, Sharma N, Ghosh M, Park YH, Jeong DK. Emerging Importance of Dietary Phytochemicals in Fight against Cancer: Role in Targeting Cancer Stem Cells. *Crit Rev Food Sci Nutr.* 2016 Feb 6:0. [Epub ahead of print]

Giovannucci E. A review of epidemiologic studies of tomatoes, lycopene, and prostate cancer. *Exp Biol Med.* (Maywood). 2002 Nov;227(10):852–9.

Sesso HD, Liu S, Gaziano JM, Buring JE. Dietary lycopene, tomato-based food products and cardiovascular disease in women. *J Nutr.* 2003 Jul;133(7):2336–41.

Feskanich D, Singh V, Willett WC, et al. Vitamin A intake and hip fractures among postmenopausal women. *JAMA.* 2002;287:47–54.

Melhus H, Michaelsson K, Kindmark A, et al. Excessive dietary intake of vitamin A is associated with reduced bone mineral density and increased risk for hip fracture. *Ann Intern Med.* 1998;129:770–8.

Food and Nutrition Board, Institute of Medicine. Dietary Reference Intakes for Vitamin A, Vitamin K, Arsenic, Boron, Chromium, Copper, Iodine, Iron, Manganese, Molybdenum, Nickel, Silicon, Vanadium, and Zinc. Washington, DC: National Academy Press, 2002. Available at *www.nap.edu.*

———. Dietary Reference Intakes for Thiamin, Riboflavin, Niacin, Vitamin B6, Folate, Vitamin B12, Pantothenic Acid, Biotin, and Choline (2000). Washington, DC: National Academy Press, 2000. Available at *http://books.nap.edu.*

Douglas RM, Chalker EB, Treacy B. Vitamin C for preventing and treating the common cold. *Cochrane Database Syst Rev.* 2000;2:CD000980.

Hemila H. Vitamin C and common cold incidence: a review of studies with subjects under heavy physical stress. *Int J Sports Med.* 1996;17:379–83.

Food and Nutrition Board, Institute of Medicine. Dietary Reference Intakes for Vitamin C, Vitamin E, Selenium, and Carotenoids. Washington, DC: National Academy Press, 2000. Available at *www.nap.edu*.

Bischoff-Ferrari HA, Willett WC, Wong JB, et al. Fracture prevention with vitamin D supplementation: a meta-analysis of randomized controlled trials. *JAMA.* 2005;293:2257–64.

Dawson-Hughes B, Heaney RP, Holick MF, et al. Estimates of optimal vitamin D status. *Osteoporos Int.* 2005;16:713–6.

Food and Nutrition Board, Institute of Medicine. Dietary Reference Intakes for Calcium, Phosphorus, Magnesium, Vitamin D, and Fluoride. Washington, DC: National Academy Press, 1999. Available at *http://books.nap.edu*.

————. Dietary Reference Intakes for Vitamin A, Vitamin K, Arsenic, Boron, Chromium, Copper, Iodine, Iron, Manganese, Molybdenum, Nickel, Silicon, Vanadium, and Zinc. Washington, DC: National Academy Press, 2002. Available at *www.nap.edu*.

Kelly GS. Nutritional and botanical interventions to assist with the adaptation to stress. *Altern Med Rev.* 1999 Aug;4(4):249–65.

Kimmatkar N, Thawani V, Hingorani L, et al. Efficacy and tolerability of Boswellia serrata extract in treatment of osteoarthritis of knee—a randomized double blind placebo controlled trial. *Phytomedicine.* 2003;10:3–7.

Sander O, Herborn G, Rau R. [Is H15 (resin extract of Boswellia serrata, "incense") a useful supplement to established drug therapy of chronic polyarthritis? Results of a double-blind pilot study]. [Article in German]. *Z Rheumatol.* 1998;57:11–6.

Mikhaeil BR, Maatoog GT, Badria FA, Amer MM. Chemistry and immuno-modulatory activity of frankincense oil. *Z Naturforsch C.* 2003;58:230–8.

Sengupta K, Alluri KV, Satish AR, et al. A double blind, randomized, placebo controlled study of the efficacy and safety of 5-Loxin for treatment of osteoarthritis of the knee. *Arthritis Res Ther.* 2008;10(4):R85. Epub 2008 Jul 30.

Piscoya J, Rodriguez Z, Bustamante SA, et al. Efficacy and safety of freeze-dried cat's claw in osteoarthritis of the knee: mechanisms of action of the species Uncaria guianensis. *Inflamm Res.* 2001;50:442–448.

Chrubasik S, Eisenberg E, Balan E, et al. Treatment of low back pain exacerbations with willow bark extract: a randomized double-blind study. *Am J Med.* 2000;109:9–14.

Braham R, Dawson B, Goodman C. The effect of glucosamine supplementation on people experiencing regular knee pain. *Br J Sports Med.* 2003;37:45–9.

Houpt JB, McMillan R, Wein C, et al. Effect of glucosamine hydrochloride in the treatment of pain of osteoarthritis of the knee. *J Rheumatol.* 1999;26:2423–30.

Wu D, Huang Y, Gu Y, Fan W. Efficacies of different preparations of glucosamine for the treatment of osteoarthritis: a meta-analysis of randomised,double-blind, placebo-controlled trials. *Int J Clin Pract.* 2013;67(6):585–94.

Clegg DO, Reda DJ, Harris CL, et al. Glucosamine, chondroitin sulfate, and the two in combination for painful knee osteoarthritis. *N Engl J Med.* 2006;354:795–808.

Uebelhart D, Thonar EJ, Delmas PD, et al. Effects of oral chondroitin sulfate on the progression of knee osteoarthritis: a pilot study. *Osteoarthritis Cartilage.* 1998;6:39–46.

Bourgeois P, Chales G, Dehais J, et al. Efficacy and tolerability of chondroitin sulfate 1200 mg/day vs chondroitin sulfate 3 x 400 mg/day vs placebo. *Osteoarthritis Cartilage.* 1998;6:25–30.

Mazieres B, Combe B, Phan Van A, et al. Chondroitin sulfate in osteoarthritis of the knee: a prospective, double blind, placebo controlled multicenter clinical study. *J Rheumatol.* 2001;28:173–81.

Usha PR, Naidu MUR. Randomised, double-blind, parallel, placebo-controlled study of oral glucosamine, methylsulfonylmethane and their combinations. *Clin Drug Invest.* 2004;24:353–63.

Kim LS, Axelrod LJ, Howard P, et al. Efficacy of methylsulfonylmethane (MSM) in osteoarthritis pain of the knee: a pilot clinical trial. *Osteoarthritis Cartilage.* 2006;14:286–94.

Barrager E, Veltmann JR Jr, Schauss AG, et al. A multicentered, open-label trial on the safety and efficacy of methylsulfonylmethane in the treatment of seasonal allergic rhinitis. *J Altern Complement Med.* 2002;8:167–73.

Caceres DD, Hancke JL, Burgos RA, et al. Prevention of common colds with Andrographis Paniculata dried extract: a pilot, double-blind trial. *Phytomedicine.* 1997;4:101–4.

Melchoir J, Spasov AA, Ostrovskij OV, et al. Double-blind, placebo-controlled pilot and phase III study of activity of standardized Andrographis paniculata Herba Nees extract fixed combination (Kan Jang) in the treatment of uncomplicated upper-respiratory tract infection. *Phytomedicine.* 2000;7:341–50.

Upton R, ed. Astragalus Root: Analytical, quality control, and therapeutic monograph. Santa Cruz, CA: *American Herbal Pharmacopoeia.* 1999:1–25.

Zakay-Rones Z, Thom E, Wollan T, et al. Randomized study of the efficacy and safety of oral elderberry extract in the treatment of influenza A and B virus infections. *J Int Med Res.* 2004;32:132–40.

Mohanty NK, Saxena S, Singh UP, et al. Lycopene as a chemopreventive agent in the treatment of high-grade prostate intraepithelial neoplasia. *Urol Oncol.* 2005;23:383–5.

Kucuk O, Sarkar FH, Sakr W, et al. Phase II randomized clinical trial of lycopene supplementation before radical prostatectomy. *Cancer Epidemiol Biomarkers Prev.* 2001;10:861–8.

Giovannucci E, Rimm EB, Liu Y, et al. A prospective study of tomato products, lycopene, and prostate cancer risk. *J Natl Cancer Inst.* 2002;94:391–8.

Forbes K, Gillette K, Sehgal I. Lycopene increases urokinase receptor and fails to inhibit growth or connexin expression in a metastatically passaged prostate cancer cell line: a brief communication. *Exp Biol Med.* (Maywood) 2003;228:967–71.

Berges RR, Windeler J, Trampisch HJ, et al. Randomised, placebo-controlled, double-blind clinical trial of beta-sitosterol in patients with benign prostatic hyperplasia. Beta-sitosterol Study Group. *Lancet.* 1995;345:1529–32.

Klippel KF, Hiltl DM, Schipp B. A multicentric, placebo-controlled, double-blind clinical trial of beta-sitosterol (phytosterol) for the treatment of benign prostatic hyperplasia. *Br J Urol.* 1997;80:427–32.

Wilt TJ, Ishani A, Stark G, et al. Saw palmetto extracts for treatment of benign prostatic hyperplasia: a systematic review. *JAMA.* 1998;280:1604–9.

Duffield-Lillico AJ, Dalkin BL, Reid ME, et al. Nutritional Prevention of Cancer Study Group. Selenium supplementation, baseline plasma selenium status and incidence of prostate cancer: an analysis of the complete treatment period of the Nutritional Prevention of Cancer Trial. *BJU Int.* 2003 May;91(7):608–12.

Chapter 6. The Orange FLOW

Cummings DE, Overduin J. Gastrointestinal regulation of food intake. *J Clin Invest.* 2007 Jan;117(1):13–23.

Avau B, Depoortere I. The bitter truth about bitter taste receptors: beyond sensing bitter in the oral cavity. *Acta Physiol.* (Oxf). 2016 Apr;216(4):407–20. doi: 10.1111/apha.12621. Epub 2015 Nov 16.

Kiecolt-Glaser JK, Jaremka L, Andridge R, Peng J, Habash D, Fagundes CP, Glaser R, Malarkey WB, Belury MA. Marital discord, past depression, and metabolic responses to high-fat meals: Interpersonal pathways to obesity. *Psychoneuroendocrinology.* 2015 Feb;52:239–50. doi: 10.1016/j.psyneuen.2014.11.018. Epub 2014 Dec 3.

Wang J, Ferruzzi MG, Ho L, Blount J, Janle EM, Gong B, Pan Y, Gowda GA, Raftery D, Arrieta-Cruz I, Sharma V, Cooper B, Lobo J, Simon JE, Zhang C, Cheng A, Qian X, Ono K, Teplow DB, Pavlides C, Dixon RA, Pasinetti GM. Brain-targeted proanthocyanidin metabolites for Alzheimer's disease treatment. *J Neurosci.* 2012 Apr 11;32(15):5144–50. doi: 10.1523/JNEUROSCI.6437–11.2012.

Pasinetti GM, Wang J, Ho L, Zhao W, Dubner L. Roles of resveratrol and other grape-derived polyphenols in Alzheimer's disease prevention and treatment. *Biochim Biophys Acta.* 2015 Jun;1852(6):1202–8. doi: 10.1016/j.bbadis.2014.10.006. Epub 2014 Oct 12.

Gendall KA, Joyce PR, Abbott RM. The effects of meal composition on subsequent craving and binge eating. *Addict Behav.* 1999 May–Jun;24(3):305–15.

Kokrashvili Z, Yee KK, Ilegems E, Iwatsuki K, Li Y, Mosinger B, Margolskee RF. Endocrine taste cells. *Br J Nutr.* 2014 Jun;111 Suppl 1:S23-9. doi: 10.1017/S0007114513002262. Epub 2014 Jan 2.

Lowcock EC, Cotterchio M, Boucher BA. Consumption of flaxseed, a rich source of lignans, is associated with reduced breast cancer risk. *Cancer Causes Control.* 2013 Apr;24(4):813–6. doi: 10.1007/s10552–013–0155–7. Epub 2013 Jan 25.

Ginter E, Simko V. Polyunsaturated fatty acids n-3: new data on heart disease, cancer, immune resistance and mental depression. *Bratisl Lek Listy*. 2010;111(12):680–5.

Calder PC, Yaqoob P. Omega-3 polyunsaturated fatty acids and human health outcomes. *Biofactors*. 2009 May–Jun;35(3):266–72. doi: 10.1002/biof.42.

Kris-Etherton PM, Harris WS, Appel LJ; AHA Nutrition Committee, American Heart Association. Omega-3 fatty acids and cardiovascular disease: new recommendations from the American Heart Association. *Arterioscler Thromb Vasc Biol*. 2003 Feb 1;23(2):151–2.

Khalesi S, Irwin C, Schubert M. Flaxseed consumption may reduce blood pressure: a systematic review and meta-analysis of controlled trials. *J Nutr*. 2015 Apr;145(4):758–65. doi: 10.3945/jn.114.205302. Epub 2015 Mar 4.

Prasad K. Flaxseed and cardiovascular health. *J Cardiovasc Pharmacol*. 2009 Nov;54(5):369–77. doi: 10.1097/FJC.0b013e3181af04e5.

Pullman-Mooar S, Laposata M, Lem D. Alteration of the cellular fatty acid profile and the production of eicosanoids in human monocytes by gamma-linolenic acid. *Arthritis Rheum*. 1990;33:1526–33.

Leventhal LJ, Boyce EG, Zurier RB. Treatment of rheumatoid arthritis with gammalinolenic acid. *Ann Intern Med*. 1993;119:867–73.

Belch J, Hill A. Evening primrose oil and borage oil in rheumatologic conditions. *Am J Clin Nutr*. 2000;71:352S–6S.

De Souza MC, Walker AF, Robinson PA, et al. A synergistic effect of a daily supplement for 1 month of 200 mg magnesium plus 50 mg vitamin B6 for the relief of anxiety-related premenstrual symptoms: a randomized, double-blind, crossover study. *J Women's Health Gend Based Med*. 2000;9:131–9.

Sharma P, Kulshreshtha S, Singh GM, et al. Role of bromocriptine and pyridoxine in premenstrual tension syndrome. *Indian J Physiol Pharmacol*. 2007 Oct–Dec;51(4):368–74.

Brush MG, Bennett T, Hansen K. Pyridoxine in the treatment of premenstrual syndrome: a retrospective survey in 630 patients. *Br J Clin Pract*. 1988 Nov;42(11):448–52.

Food and Nutrition Board, Institute of Medicine. Dietary Reference Intakes for Vitamin C, Vitamin E, Selenium, and Carotenoids. Washington, DC: National Academy Press, 2000. Available at *www.nap.edu*.

Ward MW, Holimon TD. Calcium treatment for premenstrual syndrome. *Ann Pharmacother.* 1999 Dec;33(12):1356–8.

Bertone-Johnson ER, Hankinson SE, Bendich A, et al. Calcium and vitamin D intake and risk of incident premenstrual syndrome. *Arch Intern Med.* 2005 Jun 13;165(11):1246–52.

Saeedian Kia A, Amani R, Cheraghian B. The Association between the Risk of Premenstrual Syndrome and Vitamin D, Calcium, and Magnesium Status among University Students: A Case Control Study. *Health Promot Perspect.* 2015 Oct 25;5(3):225–30. doi: 10.15171/hpp.2015.027. eCollection 2015.

Thys-Jacobs S, Ceccarelli S, Bierman A, et al. Calcium supplementation in premenstrual syndrome: a randomized crossover trial. *J Gen Intern Med.* 1989 May–Jun;4(3):183–9.

Facchinetti F, Borella P, Sances G, et al. Oral magnesium successfully relieves premenstrual mood changes. *Obstet Gynecol.* 1991;78:177–81.

Walker AF, De Souza MC, Vickers MF, et al. Magnesium supplementation alleviates premenstrual symptoms of fluid retention. *J Women's Health.* 1998;7:1157–65.

Quaranta S, Buscaglia MA, Meroni MG, et al. Pilot study of the efficacy and safety of a modified-release magnesium 250 mg tablet (Sincromag) for the treatment of premenstrual syndrome. *Clin Drug Investig.* 2007;27(1):51–8.

Reid ME, Duffield-Lillico AJ, Slate E, et al. The nutritional prevention of cancer: 400 mcg per day selenium treatment. *Nutr Cancer.* 2008 Mar–Apr;60(2):155–63.

Hess MJ, Hess PE, Sullivan MR, et al. Evaluation of cranberry tablets for the prevention of urinary tract infections in spinal cord injured patients with neurogenic bladder. *Spinal Cord.* 2008 Sep;46(9):622–6. Epub 2008 Apr 8.

Shams T, Setia MS, Hemmings R, et al. Efficacy of black cohosh-containing preparations on menopausal symptoms: a meta-analysis. *Altern Ther Health Med.* 2010;16:36–44.

Minich DM, Bland JS. A review of the clinical efficacy and safety of cruciferous vegetable phytochemicals. *Nutr Rev.* 2007 Jun;65(6 Pt 1):259–67.

Bell MC, Crowley-Nowick P, Bradlow HL, et al. Placebo-controlled trial of indole-3-carbinol in the treatment of CIN. *Gynecol Oncol.* 2000;78:123–9.

van de Weijer P, Barentsen R. Isoflavones from red clover (Promensil) significantly reduce menopausal hot flush symptoms compared with placebo. *Maturitas.* 2002;42:187–93.

Nelsen J, Barrette E, Tsouronix C, et al. Red clover (Trifolium pratense) monograph: A clinical decision support tool. *J Herb Pharmacother.* 2002;2:49–72.

Kim HJ, Kim HY, Lee SY, Seo JH, Lee E, Hong SJ. Clinical efficacy and mechanism of probiotics in allergic diseases. *Korean J Pediatr.* 2013 Sep;56(9):369–76. doi: 10.3345/kjp.2013.56.9.369. Epub 2013 Sep 30.

Ozdemir O. Various effects of different probiotic strains in allergic disorders: an update from laboratory and clinical data. *Clin Exp Immunol.* 2010 Jun;160(3):295–304. doi: 10.1111/j.1365-2249.2010.04109.x. Epub 2010 Mar 16.

Lomax AR, Calder PC. Probiotics, immune function, infection and inflammation: a review of the evidence from studies conducted in humans. *Curr Pharm Des.* 2009;15(13):1428–518.

Florowska A, Krygier K, Florowski T, Dłużewska E. Prebiotics as functional food ingredients preventing diet-related diseases. *Food Funct.* 2016 Mar 10. [Epub ahead of print]

Sabater-Molina M, Larqué E, Torrella F, Zamora S. Dietary fructooligosaccharides and potential benefits on health. *J Physiol Biochem.* 2009 Sep;65(3):315–28.

Chew BP, Wong MW, Park JS, et al. Dietary beta-carotene and astaxanthin but not canthaxanthin stimulate splenocyte function in mice. *Anticancer Res.* 1999;19;5223–8.

Omenn GS, Goodman GE, Thornquist MD, Balmes J, Cullen MR, Glass A, Keogh JP, Meyskens FL Jr, Valanis B, Williams JH Jr, Barnhart S, Cherniack MG, Brodkin CA, Hammar S. Risk factors for lung cancer and for intervention effects in CARET, the Beta-Carotene and Retinol Efficacy Trial. *J Natl Cancer Inst.* 1996 Nov 6;88(21):1550–9.

Goralczyk R. Beta-carotene and lung cancer in smokers: review of hypotheses and status of research. *Nutr Cancer.* 2009;61(6):767–74.

Chapter 7. *The Yellow FIRE*

Ludwig DS. The glycemic index: physiological mechanisms relating to obesity, diabetes, and cardiovascular disease. *JAMA.* 2002 May 8;287(18):2414–23.

Livesey G, Taylor R, Hulshof T, Howlett J. Glycemic response and health— a systematic review and meta-analysis: relations between dietary glycemic properties and health outcomes. *Am J Clin Nutr.* 2008 Jan;87(1): 258S–268S.

Ford H, Frost G. Glycaemic index, appetite and body weight. *Proc Nutr Soc.* 2010 May;69(2):199–203. doi: 10.1017/S0029665110000091.

Food and Nutrition Board, Institute of Medicine. Dietary Reference Intakes for Thiamin, Riboflavin, Niacin, Vitamin B6, Folate, Vitamin B12, Pantothenic Acid, Biotin, and Choline (2000). Washington, DC: National Academy Press, 2000. Available at: *http://books.nap.edu.*

Althius MD, Jordon NE, Ludington EA, et al. Glucose and insulin responses to dietary chromium supplements: a meta-analysis. *Am J Clin Nutr.* 2002;76:148–55.

Anton SD, Morrison CD, Cefalu WT, et al. Effects of chromium picolinate on food intake and satiety. *Diabetes Technol Ther.* 2008 Oct;10(5): 405–12.

Konrad T, Vicini P, Kusterer K, et al. Alpha-lipoic acid treatment decreases serum lactate and pyruvate concentrations and improves glucose effectiveness in lean and obese patients with Type-2 diabetes. *Diabetes Care.* 1999;22:280–7.

Kamenova P. Improvement of insulin sensitivity in patients with type-2 diabetes mellitus after oral administration of alpha-lipoic acid. *Hormones* (Athens). 2006 Oct–Dec;5(4):251–8.

Jacob S, Ruus P, Hermann R, et al. Oral administration of RAC-alpha-lipoic acid modulates insulin sensitivity in patients with type-2 diabetes mellitus: a placebo-controlled pilot trial. *Free Radic Biol Med.* 1999 Aug;27(3–4):309–14.

Khan A, Safdar M, Ali Khan M, et al. Cinnamon improves glucose and lipids of people with type-2 diabetes. *Diabetes Care.* 2003;26:3215–8.

Momordica charantia (bitter melon). Monograph. Altern Med Rev. 2007 Dec;12(4):360–3.

Madar Z, Abel R, Samish S, et al. Glucose-lowering effect of fenugreek in non-insulin dependent diabetics. *Eur J Clin Nutr.* 1988;42:51–4.

Gupta A, Gupta R, Lal B. Effect of Trigonella foenum-graecum (fenugreek) seeds on glycaemic control and insulin resistance in type-2 diabetes mellitus: a double blind placebo controlled study. *J Assoc Physicians India.* 2001;49:1057–61.

Shanmugasundaram ER, Rajeswari G, Baskaran K, et al. Use of Gymnema sylvestre leaf extract in the control of blood glucose in insulin-dependent diabetes mellitus. *J Ethnopharmacol.* 1990;30:281–94.

Baskaran K, Kizar-Ahamath B, Shanmugasundaram MR, et al. Antidiabetic effect of leaf extract from Gymnema sylvestre in non-insulin-dependent diabetes mellitus patients. *J Ethnopharmacol.* 1990;30:295–300.

Vuksan V, Sievenpiper JL, Koo VY, et al. American ginseng (Panax quinque-folius L) reduces postprandial glycemia in nondiabetic subjects and subjects with type-2 diabetes mellitus. *Arch Intern Med.* 2000;160:1009–13.

Fischer-Rasmussen W, Kjaer SK, Dahl C, et al. Ginger treatment of hyper-emesis gravidarum. *Eur J Obstet Gynecol Reprod Biol.* 1991;38:19–24.

Pongrojpaw D, Somprasit C, Chanthasenanont A. A randomized comparison of ginger and dimenhydrinate in the treatment of nausea and vomiting in pregnancy. *J Med Assoc Thai.* 2007;90:1703–9.

Wu KL, Rayner CK, Chuah SK, et al. Effects of ginger on gastric emptying and motility in healthy humans. *Eur J Gastroenterol Hepatol.* 2008 May;20(5):436–40.

Gonlachanvit S, Chen YH, Hasler WL, et al. Ginger reduces hyperglycemia-evoked gastric dysrhythmias in healthy humans: possible role of endogenous prostaglandins. *J Pharmacol Exp Ther.* 2003 Dec;307(3):1098–103. Epub 2003 Oct 8.

Prucksunand C, Indrasukhsri B, Leethochawalit M, et al. Phase II clinical trial on effect of the long turmeric (Curcuma longa Linn) on healing of peptic ulcer. *Southeast Asian J Trop Med Public Health.* 2001 Mar;32(1):208–15.

Thamlikitkul V, Bunyapraphatsara N, Dechatiwongse T, et al. Randomized double blind study of Curcuma domestica Val. for dyspepsia. *J Med Assoc Thai.* 1989;72:613–20

Yates AA, Schlicker SA, Suitor CW. Dietary reference intakes: The new basis for recommendations for calcium and related nutrients, B vitamins, and choline. *J Am Diet Assoc.* 1998;98:699–706.

Ferenci P, Dragosics B, Dittrich H, et al. Randomized controlled trial of silymarin treatment in patients with cirrhosis of the liver. *J Hepatol.* 1989;9:105–13.

Buzzelli G, Moscarella S, Giusti A, et al. A pilot study on the liver protective effect of silybin-phosphatidylcholine complex (IdB1016) in chronic active hepatitis. *Int J Clin Pharmacol Ther Toxicol.* 1993;31:456–60.

Malaguarnera M, Cammalleri L, Gargante MP, et al. L-Carnitine treatment reduces severity of physical and mental fatigue and increases cognitive functions in centenarians: a randomized and controlled clinical trial. *Am J Clin Nutr.* 2007;86:1738–44.

Dulloo AG, Duret C, Rohrer D, et al. Efficacy of a green tea extract rich in catechin polyphenols and caffeine in increasing 24-h energy expenditure and fat oxidation in humans. *Am J Clin Nutr.* 1999;70:1040–5.

Zheng G, Sayama K, Okubo T, et al. Anti-obesity effects of three major components of green tea, catechins, caffeine and theanine, in mice. *In Vivo.* 2004;18:55–62.

Venables MC, Hulston CJ, Cox HR, et al. Green tea extract ingestion, fat oxidation, and glucose tolerance in healthy humans. *Am J Clin Nutr.* 2008 Mar;87(3):778–84.

Boschmann M, Thielecke F. The effects of epigallocatechin-3-gallate on thermogenesis and fat oxidation in obese men: a pilot study. *J Am Coll Nutr.* 2007 Aug;26(4):389S–395S.

Chapter 8. The Green LOVE

McCraty, Rollin. *The Energetic Heart: Bioelectromagnetic Interactions Within and Between People.* Institute of HeartMath, 2003. Accessed 6/17/2017 at *http://store.heartmath.org/s.nl/it.A/id.617/.f*

McCraty R, Shaffer F. Heart Rate Variability: New Perspectives on Physiological Mechanisms, Assessment of Self-regulatory Capacity, and Health risk. *Glob Adv Health Med.* 2015 Jan;4(1):46–61. doi: 10.7453/gahmj.2014.073.

Shaffer F, McCraty R, Zerr CL. A healthy heart is not a metronome: an integrative review of the heart's anatomy and heart rate variability. *Front Psychol.* 2014 Sep 30;5:1040. doi: 10.3389/fpsyg.2014.01040. eCollection 2014.

Dossey, Larry. Compassion. *Explore: The Journal of Science and Healing* 2007; 3(1):1–5. Accessed 6/17/2017 at *http://www.explorejournal.com/article/S1550-8307(06)00413-7/fulltext*

Percival J, Donovan J, Kessler D, Turner K. "She believed in me." What patients with depression value in their relationship with practitioners. A secondary analysis of multiple qualitative data sets. *Health Expect.* 2016 Feb 18. doi: 10.1111/hex.12436. [Epub ahead of print]

Longmore M. Compassion as powerful as medicine. *Nurs N Z.* 2015 Oct;21(9):43.

Christakis NA, Fowler JH. The spread of obesity in a large social network over 32 years. *N Engl J Med.* 2007;357(4):370–9.

Jarman M, Ogden J, Inskip H, Lawrence W, Baird J, Cooper C, Robinson S, Barker M. How do mothers manage their preschool children's eating habits and does this change as children grow older? A longitudinal analysis. *Appetite.* 2015 Dec;95:466–74. doi: 10.1016/j.appet.2015.08.008. Epub 2015 Aug 10.

Amianto F, Ercole R, Marzola E, Abbate Daga G, Fassino S. Parents' personality clusters and eating disordered daughters' personality and psychopathology. *Psychiatry Res.* 2015 Nov 30;230(1):19–27. doi: 10.1016/j.psychres.2015.07.048. Epub 2015 Aug 6.

Lewis S, Katsikitis M, Mulgrew K. Like mother, like daughter? An examination of the emotive responses to food. *J Health Psychol.* 2015 Jun;20(6):828–38. doi: 10.1177/1359105315573442.

Gerrard, Don. *One Bowl: A Guide to Eating for Body and Spirit.* Boston: Da Capo Press, 2001.

Walsh MC, Brennan L, Pujos-Guillot E, Sébédio JL, Scalbert A, Fagan A, Higgins DG, Gibney MJ. Influence of acute phytochemical intake on human urinary metabolomic profiles. *Am J Clin Nutr.* 2007;86(6):1687–93.

Lin KH, Hsu CY, Huang YP, Lai JY, Hsieh WB, Huang MY, Yang CM, Chao PY. Chlorophyll-related compounds inhibit cell adhesion and inflammation in human aortic cells. *J Med Food.* 2013 Oct;16(10):886–98. doi: 10.1089/jmf.2012.2558. Epub 2013 Sep 25.

Yin LM, Jiang HF, Wang X, Qian XD, Gao RL, Lin XJ, Chen XH, Wang LC. Effects of sodium copper chlorophyllin on mesenchymal stem cell function in aplastic anemia mice. *Chin J Integr Med.* 2013 May;19(5):360–6. doi: 10.1007/s11655-012-1210-z. Epub 2012 Sep 21.

Hsu CY, Yang CM, Chen CM, Chao PY, Hu SP. Effects of chlorophyll-related compounds on hydrogen peroxide induced DNA damage within human lymphocytes. *J Agric Food Chem.* 2005 Apr 6;53(7):2746–50.

Hambrecht R, Hilbrich L, Erbs S, et al. Correction of endothelial dysfunction in chronic heart failure: additional effects of exercise training and oral L-arginine supplementation. *J Am Coll Cardiol.* 2000;35:706–13.

Rector TS, Bank AJ, Mullen KA, et al. Randomized, double-blind, placebo-controlled study of supplemental oral L-arginine in patients with heart failure. *Circulation.* 1996;93:2135–41.

Anderson JW, Johnstone BM, Cook-Newell ME. Meta-analysis of the effects of soy protein intake on serum lipids. *N Engl J Med.* 1995;333:276–82.

Rebholz CM, Reynolds K, Wofford MR, Chen J, Kelly TN, Mei H, Whelton PK, He J. Effect of soybean protein on novel cardiovascular disease risk factors: a randomized controlled trial. *Eur J Clin Nutr.* 2013 Jan;67(1):58–63. doi: 10.1038/ejcn.2012.186. Epub 2012 Nov 28.

Bakhtiary A, Yassin Z, Hanachi P, Rahmat A, Ahmad Z, Jalali F. Effects of soy on metabolic biomarkers of cardiovascular disease in elderly women with metabolic syndrome. *Arch Iran Med.* 2012 Aug;15(8):462–8. doi: 012158/AIM.004.

Nechuta SJ, Caan BJ, Chen WY, Lu W, Chen Z, Kwan ML, Flatt SW, Zheng Y, Zheng W, Pierce JP, Shu XO. Soy food intake after diagnosis of breast cancer and survival: an in-depth analysis of combined evidence from cohort studies of US and Chinese women. *Am J Clin Nutr.* 2012 Jul;96(1):123–32. doi: 10.3945/ajcn.112.035972. Epub 2012 May 30.

Fritz H, Seely D, Flower G, Skidmore B, Fernandes R, Vadeboncoeur S, Kennedy D, Cooley K, Wong R, Sagar S, Sabri E, Fergusson D. Soy, red clover, and isoflavones and breast cancer: a systematic review. *PLoS One.* 2013 Nov 28;8(11):e81968. doi: 10.1371/journal.pone.0081968. eCollection 2013.

Thomas AJ, Ismail R, Taylor-Swanson L, Cray L, Schnall JG, Mitchell ES, Woods NF. Effects of isoflavones and amino acid therapies for hot flashes and co-occurring symptoms during the menopausal transition and early postmenopause: a systematic review. *Maturitas.* 2014 Aug;78(4):263–76. doi: 10.1016/j.maturitas.2014.05.007. Epub 2014 May 28.

Wei P, Liu M, Chen Y, Chen DC. Systematic review of soy isoflavone supplements on osteoporosis in women. *Asian Pac J Trop Med.* 2012 Mar;5(3):243–8. doi: 10.1016/S1995-7645(12)60033-9.

van der Griend R, Biesma DH, Haas FJLM, et al. The effect of different treatment regimens in reducing fasting and postmethionine-load homocysteine concentrations. *J Int Med.* 2000;248:223–9.

van der Griend R, Haas FJ, Biesma DH, et al. Combination of low-dose folic acid and pyridoxine for treatment of hyperhomocysteinaemia in patients with premature arterial disease and their relatives. *Atherosclerosis*. 1999;143:177–83.

Cheung AM, Tile L, Lee Y, et al. Vitamin K supplementation in postmenopausal women with osteopenia (ECKO trial): a randomized controlled trial. *PLoS Med*. 2008 Oct 14;5(10):e196.

Olson RE. Osteoporosis and vitamin K intake. *Am J Clin Nutr*. 2000;71:1031–2.

Patrick L. Iodine: deficiency and therapeutic considerations. *Altern Med Rev*. 2008 Jun;13(2):116–27.

Ghent WR, Eskin BA, Low DA, et al. Iodine replacement in fibrocystic disease of the breast. *Can J Surg*. 1993;36:453–60.

Sanjuliani AF, de Abreu Fagundes VG, Francischetti EA. Effects of magnesium on blood pressure and intracellular ion levels of Brazilian hypertensive patients. *Int J Cardiol*. 1996;56:177–83.

Widman L, Wester PO, Stegmayr BK, et al. The dose-dependent reduction in blood pressure through administration of magnesium. A double blind placebo controlled cross-over study. *Am J Hypertens*. 1993;6:41–5.

Jee SH, Miller ER III, Guallar E, et al. The effect of magnesium supplementation on blood pressure: a meta-analysis of randomized clinical trials. *Am J Hypertens*. 2002;15:691–6.

Guerrero-Romero F, Rodríguez-Morán M. The effect of lowering blood pressure by magnesium supplementation in diabetic hypertensive adults with low serum magnesium levels: a randomized, double-blind, placebo-controlled clinical trial. *J Hum Hypertens*. 2008 Nov 20. [Epub ahead of print]

Food and Drug Administration. FDA Talk Paper: FDA Authorizes New Coronary Heart Disease Health Claim for Plant Sterol and Plant Stanol Esters. September 5, 2000. Accessed 11/21/08 at *www.fda.gov*.

Heber D, Yip I, Ashley JM, et al. Cholesterol-lowering effects of a proprietary Chinese red-yeast-rice dietary supplement. *Am J Clin Nutr*. 1999;69:231–6.

Huang CF, Li TC, Lin CC, et al. Efficacy of Monascus purpureus Went rice on lowering lipid ratios in hypercholesterolemic patients. *Eur J Cardiovasc Prev Rehabil*. 2007 Jun;14(3):438–40.

Anonymous. Quercetin. *Alt Med Rev*. 1998;3:140–3.

Edwards RL, Lyon T, Litwin SE, et al. Quercetin reduces blood pressure in hypertensive subjects. *J Nutr*. 2007 Nov;137(11):2405–11.

Belcaro G, Cesarone MR, Ledda A, et al. 5-Year control and treatment of edema and increased capillary filtration in venous hypertension and diabetic microangiopathy using O-(beta-hydroxyethyl)-rutosides: a prospective comparative clinical registry. *Angiology*. 2008 Feb-Mar;59 Suppl 1:14S–20S.

Ried K, Frank OR, Stocks NP, et al. Effect of garlic on blood pressure: A systematic review and meta-analysis. *BMC Cardiovasc Disord*. 2008;8:13.

Koscielny J, Klüssendorf D, Latza R, et al. The antiatherosclerotic effect of Allium sativum. *Atherosclerosis*. 1999;144:237–49.

De Sanctis MT, Belcaro G, Incandela L, et al. Treatment of edema and increased capillary filtration in venous hypertension with total triterpenic fraction of Centella asiatica: a clinical, prospective, placebo-controlled, randomized, dose-ranging trial. *Angiology*. 2001;52 Suppl 2:S55–9

Suter A, Bommer S, Rechner J. Treatment of patients with venous insufficiency with fresh plant horse chestnut seed extract: a review of 5 clinical studies. *Adv Ther*. 2006 Jan–Feb;23(1):179–90.

Tauchert M. Efficacy and safety of crataegus extract WS 1442 in comparison with placebo in patients with chronic stable New York Heart Association class-III heart failure. *Am Heart J*. 2002;143:910–5.

Holubarsch CJ, Colucci WS, Meinertz T, et al. The efficacy and safety of Crataegus extract WS(R) 1442 in patients with heart failure: The SPICE trial. *Eur J Heart Fail*. 2008 Nov 17. [Epub ahead of print]

Sesso HD, Buring JE, Norkus EP, et al. Plasma lycopene, other carotenoids, and retinol and the risk of cardiovascular disease in women. *Am J Clin Nutr*. 2004 Jan;79(1):47–53.

Sesso HD, Liu S, Gaziano JM, et al. Dietary lycopene, tomato-based food products and cardiovascular disease in women. *J Nutr*. 2003;133:2336–41.

Neuman I, Nahum H, Ben-Amotz A. Reduction of exercise-induced asthma oxidative stress by lycopene, a natural antioxidant. *Allergy*. 2000;55:1184–9.

Chapter 9. The Aquamarine TRUTH

Blondin SA, Anzman-Frasca S, Djang HC, Economos CD. Breakfast consumption and adiposity among children and adolescents: an updated review of the literature. *Pediatr Obes*. 2016 Feb 4. doi: 10.1111 /ijpo.12082. [Epub ahead of print]

Hoch SJ, Bradlow EL, Wansink B. The variety of assortment. *Marketing Science.* 1999; 18(4): 527–46.

Kahn BE, Wansink B. The influence of assortment structure on perceived variety and consumption quantities. *Journal of Consumer Research.* 2004; 30(4):519–33.

Patrick L. Iodine: deficiency and therapeutic considerations. *Altern Med Rev.* 2008 Jun;13(2):116–27.

Mazokopakis EE, Papadakis JA, Papadomanolaki MG, et al. Effects of 12 months treatment with L-selenomethionine on serum anti-TPO Levels in Patients with Hashimoto's thyroiditis. *Thyroid.* 2007 Jul;17(7):609–12.

Allergic sinusitis. MedlinePlus Medical Encyclopedia. Accessed 11/21/08 at *www.nlm.nih.gov.*

Thornhill SM, Kelly AM. Natural treatment of perennial allergic rhinitis. *Altern Med Rev.* 2000 Oct;5(5):448–54.

Mao TK, Van de Water J, Gershwin ME. Effects of a Spirulina-based dietary supplement on cytokine production from allergic rhinitis patients. *J Med Food.* 2005;8:27–30.

Mittman P. Randomized, double-blind study of freeze-dried Urtica dioica in the treatment of allergic rhinitis. *Planta Med.* 1990;56:44–7.

Thie NM, Prasad NG, Major PW. Evaluation of glucosamine sulfate compared to ibuprofen for the treatment of temporomandibular joint osteo-arthritis: a randomized double blind controlled 3-month clinical trial. *J Rheumatol.* 2001;28:1347–55.

Attias J, Weisz G, Almog S, et al. Oral magnesium intake reduces permanent hearing loss induced by noise exposure. *Am J Otolaryngol.* 1994 Jan–Feb;15(1):26–32.

Nageris BI, Ulanovski D, Attias J. Magnesium treatment for sudden hearing loss. *Ann Otol Rhinol Laryngol.* 2004 Aug;113(8):672–5.

Heyneman CA. Zinc deficiency and taste disorders. *Ann Pharmacother.* 1996;30:186–7.

Chapter 10. The Indigo INSIGHT

Avallone R, Zanoli P, Puia G, Kleinschnitz M, Schreier P, Baraldi M. Pharmacological profile of apigenin, a flavonoid isolated from Matricaria chamomilla. *Biochem Pharmacol.* 2000 Jun 1;59(11):1387–94.

Campbell EL, Chebib M, Johnston GA. The dietary flavonoids apigenin and (-)-epigallocatechin gallate enhance the positive modulation by diazepam of the activation by GABA of recombinant GABA(A) receptors. *Biochem Pharmacol*. 2004 Oct 15;68(8):1631–8.

Cho S, Park JH, Pae AN, Han D, Kim D, Cho NC, No KT, Yang H, Yoon M, Lee C, Shimizu M, Baek NI. Hypnotic effects and GABAergic mechanism of licorice (Glycyrrhiza glabra) ethanol extract and its major flavonoid constituent glabrol. *Bioorg Med Chem*. 2012 Jun 1;20(11):3493–501. doi: 10.1016/j.bmc.2012.04.011. Epub 2012 Apr 11.

Jäger AK, Saaby L. Flavonoids and the CNS. *Molecules*. 2011 Feb 10;16(2):1471–85. doi: 10.3390/molecules16021471.

Kavvadias D, Monschein V, Sand P, Riederer P, Schreier P. Constituents of sage (Salvia officinalis) with in vitro affinity to human brain benzodiazepine receptor. *Planta Med*. 2003 Feb;69(2):113–7.

Nielsen M, Frøkjaer S, Braestrup C. High affinity of the naturally-occurring biflavonoid, amentoflavon, to brain benzodiazepine receptors in vitro. *Biochem Pharmacol*. 1988 Sep 1;37(17):3285–7.

Medina JH, Paladini AC, Wolfman C, Levi de Stein M, Calvo D, Diaz LE, Peña C. Chrysin (5,7-di-OH-flavone), a naturally-occurring ligand for benzodiazepine receptors, with anticonvulsant properties. *Biochem Pharmacol*. 1990 Nov 15;40(10):2227–31.

Salgueiro JB, Ardenghi P, Dias M, Ferreira MB, Izquierdo I, Medina JH. Anxiolytic natural and synthetic flavonoid ligands of the central benzodiazepine receptor have no effect on memory tasks in rats. *Pharmacol Biochem Behav*. 1997 Dec;58(4):887–91.

Viola H, Wasowski C, Levi de Stein M, Wolfman C, Silveira R, Dajas F, Medina JH, Paladini AC. Apigenin, a component of Matricaria recutita flowers, is a central benzodiazepine receptors-ligand with anxiolytic effects. *Planta Med*. 1995 Jun;61(3):213–16.

Wolfman C, Viola H, Paladini A, Dajas F, Medina JH. Possible anxiolytic effects of chrysin, a central benzodiazepine receptor ligand isolated from Passiflora coerulea. *Pharmacol Biochem Behav*. 1994 Jan;47(1):1–4.

Macdiarmid JI, Hetherington MM. Mood modulation by food: an exploration of affect and cravings in "chocolate addicts." *Br J Clin Psychol*. 1995;34 (Pt 1):129–38.

Michener W, Rozin P. Pharmacological versus sensory factors in the satiation of chocolate craving. *Physiol Behav*. 1994;56(3):419–22.

Sansone R, Rodriguez-Mateos A, Heuel J, Falk D, Schuler D, Wagstaff R, Kuhnle GG, Spencer JP, Schroeter H, Merx MW, Kelm M, Heiss C; Flaviola Consortium, European Union 7th Framework Program. Cocoa flavanol intake improves endothelial function and Framingham Risk Score in healthy men and women: a randomised, controlled, double-masked trial: the Flaviola Health Study. *Br J Nutr*. 2015 Oct 28;114(8):1246–55. doi: 10.1017/S0007114515002822. Epub 2015 Sep 9.

Ng TP, Chiam PC, Lee T, Chua HC, Lim L, Kua EH. Curry consumption and cognitive function in the elderly. *Am J Epidemiol*. 2006 Nov 1;164(9):898–906. Epub 2006 Jul 26.

Ringman JM, Frautschy SA, Cole GM, Masterman DL, Cummings JL. A potential role of the curry spice curcumin in Alzheimer's disease. *Curr Alzheimer Res*. 2005 Apr;2(2):131–6.

Shoba G, Joy D, Joseph T, Majeed M, Rajendran R, Srinivas PS. Influence of piperine on the pharmacokinetics of curcumin in animals and human volunteers. *Planta Med*. 1998 May;64(4):353–6.

Puangsombat K, Jirapakkul W, Smith JS. Inhibitory activity of Asian spices on heterocyclic amines formation in cooked beef patties. *J Food Sci*. 2011 Oct;76(8):T174–80. doi: 10.1111/j.1750-3841.2011.02338.x. Epub 2011 Sep 13.

Guarrera PM, Savo V. Wild food plants used in traditional vegetable mixtures in Italy. *J Ethnopharmacol*. 2016 Mar 1. pii: S0378-8741(16)30094-0.

Aggrawal B and Yost D. *Healing Spices: How to Use 50 Everyday and Exotic Spices to Boost Health and Beat Disease*. New York: Sterling, 2011.

Holmes MV, Dale CE, Zuccolo L, Silverwood RJ, et al. Association between alcohol and cardiovascular disease: Mendelian randomisation analysis based on individual participant data. *BMJ*. 2014 Jul 10;349:g4164. doi: 10.1136/bmj.g4164.

Emsley R, Myburgh C, Oosthuizen P, et al. Randomized, placebo-controlled study of ethyl-eicosapentaenoic acid as supplemental treatment in schizophrenia. *Am J Psychiatry*. 2002;159:1596–8.

Joy CB, Mumby-Croft R, Joy LA. Polyunsaturated fatty acid supplementation for schizophrenia. *Cochrane Database Syst Rev*. 2006;3:CD001257.

Zanarini MC, Frankenburg FR. Omega-3 Fatty acid treatment of women with borderline personality disorder: a double-blind, placebo-controlled pilot study. *Am J Psychiatry*. 2003;160:167–9.

Sivrioglu EY, Kirli S, Sipahioglu D, et al. The impact of omega-3 fatty acids, vitamins E and C supplementation on treatment outcome and side effects in schizophrenia patients treated with haloperidol: an open-label pilot study. *Prog Neuropsychopharmacol Biol Psychiatry*. 2007 Oct 1;31(7):1493–9. Epub 2007 Jul 13.

Malcolm CA, McCulloch DL, Montgomery C, et al. Maternal docosahexae-noic acid supplementation during pregnancy and visual evoked potential development in term infants: a double blind, prospective, randomised trial. *Arch Dis Child Fetal Neonatal Ed*. 2003;88:F383–90.

Stordy BJ. Dark adaptation, motor skills, docosahexaenoic acid, and dyslexia. *Am J Clin Nutr*. 2000;71:323S–6S.

Lerner V, Miodownik C, Kaptsan A, et al. Vitamin B6 as add-on treatment in chronic schizophrenic and schizoaffective patients: a double-blind, placebo-controlled study. *J Clin Psychiatry*. 2002 Jan;63(1):54–8.

Wyatt KM, Dimmock PW, Jones PW, et al. Efficacy of vitamin B-6 in the treatment of premenstrual syndrome: systematic review. *BMJ*. 1999 May 22;318(7195):1375–81.

Hvas AM, Juul S, Bech P, et al. Vitamin B6 level is associated with symptoms of depression. *Psychother Psychosom*. 2004 Nov–Dec;73(6):340–3.

Kuzminski AM, Del Giacco EJ, Allen RH, et al. Effective treatment of cobalamin deficiency with oral cobalamin. *Blood*. 1998;92:1191–1198.

Andres E, Kurtz JE, Perrin AE, et al. Oral cobalamin therapy for the treatment of patients with food-cobalamin malabsorption. *Am J Med*. 2001;111:126–9.

Wald DS, Bishop L, Wald NJ, et al. Randomized trial of folic acid supplementation and serum homocysteine levels. *Arch Intern Med*. 2001;161:695–700.

Kendrick T, Dunn N, Robinson S, et al. A longitudinal study of blood folate levels and depressive symptoms among young women in the Southampton Women's Survey. *J Epidemiol Community Health*. 2008 Nov;62(11):966–72.

Tolmunen T, Hintikka J, Voutilainen S, et al. Association between depressive symptoms and serum concentrations of homocysteine in men: a population study. *Am J Clin Nutr*. 2004 Dec;80(6):1574–8.

Homocysteine Lowering Trialists' Collaboration. Dose-dependent effects of folic acid on blood concentrations of homocysteine: a meta-analysis of the randomized trials. *Am J Clin Nutr*. 2005 Oct;82(4):806–12.

Young SN. Folate and depression—a neglected problem. *J Psychiatry Neurosci.* 2007 Mar;32(2):80–2.

Cooper JR. The role of ascorbic acid in the oxidation of tryptophan to 5-hydroxytryptophan. *Ann NY Acad Sci.* 1961;92:208–11.

Milner G. Ascorbic acid in chronic psychiatric patients: a controlled trial. *Br J Psychiatry.* 1963;109:294–9.

Dakhale GN, Khanzode SD, Khanzode SS, et al. Supplementation of vitamin C with atypical antipsychotics reduces oxidative stress and improves the outcome of schizophrenia. *Psychopharmacology.* (Berl). 2005 Nov;182(4):494–8. Epub 2005 Oct 19.

Sivrioglu EY, Kirli S, Sipahioglu D, et al. The impact of omega-3 fatty acids, vitamins E and C supplementation on treatment outcome and side effects in schizophrenia patients treated with haloperidol: an open-label pilot study. *Prog Neuropsychopharmacol Biol Psychiatry.* 2007 Oct 1;31(7):1493–9. Epub 2007 Jul 13.

Przybelski RJ, Binkley NC. Is vitamin D important for preserving cognition? A positive correlation of serum 25-hydroxyvitamin D concentration with cognitive function. *Arch Biochem Biophys.* 2007 Apr 15;460(2):202–5. Epub 2007 Jan 8.

Johnson MA, Fischer JG, Park S. Vitamin D deficiency and insufficiency in the Georgia Older Americans Nutrition Program. *J Nutr Elder.* 2008;27(1–2):29–46.

Jorde R, Sneve M, Figenschau Y, et al. Effects of vitamin D supplementation on symptoms of depression in overweight and obese subjects: randomized double blind trial. *J Intern Med.* 2008 Dec 1;264(6):599–609. Epub 2008 Sep 10.

Hoogendijk WJ, Lips P, Dik MG, et al. Depression is associated with decreased 25-hydroxyvitamin D and increased parathyroid hormone levels in older adults. *Arch Gen Psychiatry.* 2008 May;65(5):508–12.

Wilkins CH, Sheline YI, Roe CM, et al. Vitamin D deficiency is associated with low mood and worse cognitive performance in older adults. *Am J Geriatr Psychiatry.* 2006 Dec;14(12):1032–40.

Donald Brown, N.D., Alan R. Gaby, M.D., and Ronald Reichert, N.D. Altering the Brain's Chemistry to Elevate Mood. Accessed 11/22/08 at *www.healthyplace.com.*

Siwek M, Wróbel A, Dudek D, et al. [The role of copper and magnesium in the pathogenesis and treatment of affective disorders] *Psychiatr Pol.* 2005 Sep–Oct;39(5):911–20.

Peikert A, Wilimzig C, Kohne-Volland R. Prophylaxis of migraine with oral magnesium: results from a prospective, multi-center, placebo-controlled and double-blind randomized study. *Cephalalgia.* 1996;16:257–63.

Held K, Antonijevic IA, Künzel H, et al. Oral Mg(2+) supplementation reverses age-related neuroendocrine and sleep EEG changes in humans. *Pharmacopsychiatry.* 2002 Jul;35(4):135–43.

Thal LJ, Carta A, Clarke WR, et al. A 1-year multicenter placebo-controlled study of acetyl-L-carnitine in patients with Alzheimer's Disease. *Neurology.* 1996;47:705–11.

Sano M, Bell K, Cote L, et al. Double-blind parallel design pilot study of acetyl levocarnitine in patients with Alzheimer's Disease. *Arch Neurol.* 1992;49:1137–41.

Rai G, Wright G, Scott L, et al. Double-blind, placebo controlled study of acetyl-l-carnitine in patients with Alzheimer's dementia. *Curr Med Res Opin.* 1990;11:638–47.

Nakajima T, Kudo Y, Kaneko Z. Clinical evaluation of 5-hydroxy-L-tryptophan as an antidepressant drug. *Folia Psychiatr Neurol Jpn.* 1978;32:223–30.

Levine J, Barak Y, Gonzalves M, et al. Double-blind, controlled trial of inositol treatment of depression. *Am J Psychiatry.* 1995;152:792–4.

Benjamin J, Levine J, Fux M, et al. Double-blind, placebo-controlled, crossover trial of inositol treatment for panic disorder. *Am J Psychiatry.* 1995;152:1084–6.

Palatnik A, Frolov K, Fux M, et al. Double-blind, controlled, crossover trial of inositol versus fluvoxamine for the treatment of panic disorder. *J Clin Psychopharmacol.* 2001;21:335–9.

Fux M, Levine J, Aviv A, et al. Inositol treatment of obsessive-compulsive disorder. *Am J Psychiatry.* 1996;153:1219–21.

Kim HL, Streltzer J, Goebert D. St. John's wort for depression: A meta analysis of well-defined clinical trials. *J Nerv Ment Dis.* 1999;187:532–9.

Linde K, Ramirez G, Mulrow CD, et al. St. John's wort for depression: an overview and meta-analysis of randomized clinical trials. *BMJ.* 1996;313:253–8.

Zhdanova IV, Wurtman RJ, Regan MM, et al. Melatonin treatment for age-related insomnia. *J Clin Endocrinol Metab.* 2001;86:4727–30.

Brusco LI, Fainstein I, Marquez M, et al. Effect of melatonin in selected populations of sleep-disturbed patients. *Biol Signals Recept.* 1999;8: 126–31.

Dorn M. [Efficacy and tolerability of Baldrian versus oxazepam in non-organic and non-psychiatric insomniacs: a randomized, double-blind, clinical, comparative study]. [Article in German]. *Forsch Komplementarmed Klass Naturheilkd.* 2000;7:79–84.

Bent S, Padula A, Moore D, et al. Valerian for sleep: a systematic review and meta-analysis. *Am J Med.* 2006 Dec;119(12):1005–12.

Richer S, Stiles W, Statkute L, et al. Double-masked, placebo-controlled, randomized trial of lutein and antioxidant supplementation in the intervention of atrophic age-related macular degermation: the Veterans LAST study (Lutein Antioxidant Supplement Trial). *Optometry.* 2004;75:216–30.

Bahrami H, Melia M, Dagnelie G. Lutein supplementation in retinitis pigmentosa: PC-based vision assessment in a randomized double-masked placebo-controlled clinical trial [NCT00029289]. *BMC Ophthalmol.* 2006 Jun 7;6:23.

Olmedilla B, Granado F, Blanco I, et al. Lutein, but not alpha-tocopherol, supplementation improves visual function in patients with age-related cataracts: a 2-year double-blind, placebo-controlled pilot study. *Nutrition.* 2003 Jan;19(1):21–4.

Stough C, Lloyd J, Clarke J, et al. The chronic effects of an extract of Bacopa monniera (Brahmi) on cognitive function in healthy human subjects. *Psychopharmacology.* 2001;156:481–4.

Stough C, Downey LA, Lloyd J, et al. Examining the nootropic effects of a special extract of Bacopa monniera on human cognitive functioning: 90-day double-blind placebo-controlled randomized trial. *Phytother Res.* 2008 Aug 6. [Epub ahead of print]

Wattanathorn J, Mator L, Muchimapura S, et al. Positive modulation of cognition and mood in the healthy elderly volunteer following the administration of Centella asiatica. *J Ethnopharmacol.* 2008 Mar 5;116(2):325–32. Epub 2007 Dec 4.

Crook T, Petrie W, Wells C, Massari DC. Effects of phosphatidylserine in Alzheimer's disease. *Psychopharmacol Bull.* 1992;28:61–6.

Delwaide PJ, Gyselynck-Mambourg AM, Hurlet A, Ylieff M. Double-blind, randomized, controlled study of phosphatidylserine in senile demented patients. *Acta Neurol Scand*. 1986;73:136–40.

Schreiber S, Kampf-Sherf O, Gorfine M, et al. An open trial of plant-source derived phosphatidylserine for treatment of age-related cognitive decline. *Isr J Psychiatry Relat Sci*. 2000;37:302–7.

Kelly SP, Gomez-Ramirez M, Montesi JL, et al. L-theanine and caffeine in combination affect human cognition as evidenced by oscillatory alpha-band activity and attention task performance. *J Nutr*. 2008 Aug;138(8):1572S–1577S.

Gomez-Ramirez M, Kelly SP, Montesi JL, et al. The Effects of L-theanine on Alpha-Band Oscillatory Brain Activity During a Visuo-Spatial Attention Task. *Brain Topogr*. 2008 Oct 9. [Epub ahead of print]

Chapter 11. The White SPIRIT

Wijk RV, Wijk EP. An introduction to human biophoton emission. *Forsch Komplementarmed Klass Naturheilkd*. 2005 Apr;12(2):77–83.

Salari V, Valian H, Bassereh H, Bókkon I, Barkhordari A.Ultraweak photon emission in the brain. *J Integr Neurosci*. 2015 Sep;14(3):419–29. doi: 10.1142/S0219635215300012. Epub 2015 Sep 4.

Brandhorst S, Choi IY, Wei M, Cheng CW, Sedrakyan S, Navarrete G, Dubeau L, Yap LP, Park R, Vinciguerra M, Di Biase S, Mirzaei H, Mirisola MG, Childress P, Ji L, Groshen S, Penna F, Odetti P, Perin L, Conti PS, Ikeno Y, Kennedy BK, Cohen P, Morgan TE, Dorff TB, Longo VD. A Periodic Diet that Mimics Fasting Promotes Multi-System Regeneration, Enhanced Cognitive Performance, and Healthspan. *Cell Metab*. 2015 Jul 7;22(1):86–99. doi: 10.1016/j.cmet.2015.05.012. Epub 2015 Jun 18.

Heilbronn LK, de Jonge L, Frisard MI, DeLany JP, Larson-Meyer DE, Rood J, Nguyen T, Martin CK, Volaufova J, Most MM, Greenway FL, Smith SR, Deutsch WA, Williamson DA, Ravussin E; Pennington CALERIE Team. Effect of 6-month calorie restriction on biomarkers of longevity, metabolic adaptation, and oxidative stress in overweight individuals: a randomized controlled trial. *JAMA*. 2006 Apr 5;295(13):1539–48.

Anderson GH, Soeandy CD, Smith CE. White vegetables: glycemia and satiety. *Adv Nutr*. 2013 May 1;4(3):356S–67S. doi: 10.3945 /an.112.003509.

Cardoso DA, Moreira AS, De Oliveira GM, Raggio Luiz R, Rosa G. A Coconut Extra Virgin Oil-Rich Diet Increases Hdl Cholesterol And Decreases Waist Circumference And Body Mass In Coronary Artery Disease Patients. *Nutr Hosp*. 2015 Nov 1;32(n05):2144–2152.

Kirsh VA, Peters U, Mayne ST, Subar AF, Chatterjee N, Johnson CC, Hayes RB; Prostate, Lung, Colorectal and Ovarian Cancer Screening Trial. Prospective study of fruit and vegetable intake and risk of prostate cancer. *J Natl Cancer Inst*. 2007 Aug 1;99(15):1200–9. Epub 2007 Jul 24.

Sharquie KE, Al-Obaidi HK. Onion juice (Allium cepa L.), a new topical treatment for alopecia areata. *J Dermatol*. 2002 Jun;29(6):343–6.

Slimestad R, Fossen T, Vågen IM. Onions: a source of unique dietary flavonoids. *J Agric Food Chem*. 2007 Dec 12;55(25):10067–80. Epub 2007 Nov 13.

Jamal GA, Carmichael H. The effect of gamma-linolenic acid on human diabetic peripheral neuropathy: a double-blind placebo-controlled trial. *Diabet Med*. 1990;7:319–23.

Keen H, Payan J, Allawi J, et al. Treatment of diabetic neuropathy with gamma-linolenic acid. The gamma-Linolenic Acid Multicenter Trial Group. *Diabetes Care*. 1993;16:8–15.

Okuda Y, Mizutani M, Ogawa M, et al. Long-term effects of eicosapentaenoic acid on diabetic peripheral neuropathy and serum lipids in patients with type-II diabetes mellitus. *J Diabetes Complications*. 1996 Sep–Oct;10(5):280–7.

Gerbi A, Maixent JM, Ansaldi JL, et al. Fish oil supplementation prevents diabetes-induced nerve conduction velocity and neuroanatomical changes in rats. *J Nutr*. 1999 Jan;129(1):207–13.

Koutsikos D, Agroyannis B, Tzanatos-Exarchou H. Biotin for diabetic peripheral neuropathy. *Biomed Pharmacother*. 1990;44(10):511–14.

Haupt E, Ledermann H, Köpcke W. Benfotiamine in the treatment of diabetic polyneuropathy--a three-week randomized, controlled pilot study (BEDIP study). *Int J Clin Pharmacol Ther*. 2005 Feb;43(2):71–7.

Stracke H, Gaus W, Achenbach U, Federlin K, Bretzel RG. Benfotiamine in diabetic polyneuropathy (BENDIP): results of a randomised, double blind, placebo-controlled clinical study. *Exp Clin Endocrinol Diabetes*. 2008 Nov;116(10):600–5. doi: 10.1055/s-2008-1065351. Epub 2008 May 13.

Scalabrino G, Peracchi M. New insights into the pathophysiology of cobalamin deficiency. *Trends Mol Med.* 2006 Jun;12(6):247–54. Epub 2006 May 11.

Head KA. Peripheral neuropathy: pathogenic mechanisms and alternative therapies. *Altern Med Rev.* 2006 Dec;11(4):294–329.

Tütüncü NB, Bayraktar M, Varli K. Reversal of defective nerve conduction with vitamin E supplementation in type-2 diabetes: a preliminary study. *Diabetes Care.* 1998 Nov;21(11):1915–8.

De Leeuw I, Engelen W, De Block C, et al. Long-term magnesium supplementation influences favourably the natural evolution of neuropathy in Mg-depleted type-1 diabetic patients (T1dm). *Magnes Res.* 2004 Jun;17(2):109–14.

Calabrese V, Scapagnini G, Ravagna A, Bella R, Butterfield DA, Calvani M, Pennisi G, Giuffrida Stella AM. Disruption of thiol homeostasis and nitrosative stress in the cerebrospinal fluid of patients with active multiple sclerosis: evidence for a protective role of acetylcarnitine. *Neurochem Res.* 2003 Sep;28(9):1321–8.

De Grandis D, Minardi C. Acetyl-L-carnitine (levacecarnine) in the treatment of diabetic neuropathy. A long-term, randomised, double-blind, placebo-controlled study. *Drugs R D.* 2002;3:223–31.

Sima AAF, Calvani M, Mehra M, et al. Acetyl-L-carnitine improves pain, nerve regeneration, and vibratory perception in patients with chronic diabetic neuropathy: An analysis of two randomized, placebo-controlled trials. *Diabetes Care.* 2005;28:89–94.

Ziegler D, Hanefeld M, Ruhnau K, et al. Treatment of symptomatic diabetic polyneuropathy with the antioxidant alpha-lipoic acid: A 7-month, multicenter, randomized, controlled trial (ALADIN III Study). *Diabetes Care.* 1999;22:1296–301.

Reljanovic M, Reichel G, Rett K, et al. Treatment of diabetic polyneuropathy with the antioxidant thioctic acid (alpha-lipoic acid): A 2-year, multicenter, randomized, double-blind, placebo-controlled trial (ALADIN II). Alpha Lipoic Acid in Diabetic Neuropathy. *Free Radic Res.* 1999;31:171–7.

Ruhnau KJ, Meissner HP, Finn JR, et al. Effects of 3-week oral treatment with the antioxidant thioctic acid (alpha-lipoic acid) in symptomatic diabetic polyneuropathy. *Diabet Med.* 1999;16:1040–3.

Shults CW, Oakes D, Kieburtz K, et al. Effects of coenzyme Q10 in early Parkinson disease: evidence of slowing of the functional decline. *Arch Neurol.* 2002;59:1541–50.

Yates AA, Schlicker SA, Suitor CW. Dietary reference intakes: The new basis for recommendations for calcium and related nutrients, B vitamins, and choline. *J Am Diet Assoc.* 1998;98:699–706.

Sima AA, Dunlap JA, Davidson EP, et al. Supplemental myo-inositol prevents L-fucose-induced diabetic neuropathy. *Diabetes.* 1997 Feb;46(2):301–6.

Sundkvist G, Dahlin LB, Nilsson H, et al. Sorbitol and myo-inositol levels and morphology of sural nerve in relation to peripheral nerve function and clinical neuropathy in men with diabetic, impaired, and normal glucose tolerance. *Diabet Med.* 2000 Apr;17(4):259–68.

Bourre JM. Effects of nutrients (in food) on the structure and function of the nervous system: update on dietary requirements for brain. Part 1: micronutrients. *J Nutr Health Aging.* 2006 Sep–Oct;10(5):377–85.

Zeisel SH. Choline: needed for normal development of memory. *J Am Coll Nutr.* 2000;19:528S–31S.

Shaw GM, Carmichael SL, Yang W, et al. Periconceptional dietary intake of choline and betaine and neural tube defects in offspring. *Am J Epidemiol.* 2004;160:102–9.

Gertz M, Nguyen GT, Fischer F, Suenkel B, Schlicker C, Fränzel B, Tomaschewski J, Aladini F, Becker C, Wolters D, Steegborn C. A molecular mechanism for direct sirtuin activation by resveratrol. *PLoS One.* 2012;7(11):e49761. doi: 10.1371/journal.pone.0049761. Epub 2012 Nov 21.

ABOUT THE AUTHOR

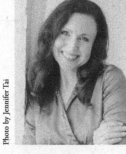

Photo by Jennifer Tai

Dr. Deanna Minich is an internationally recognized health expert and author with more than twenty years of experience in nutrition, mind-body health, and functional medicine. Dr. Minich holds master's and doctoral degrees in nutrition and has lectured extensively throughout the world on health topics, teaching patients and health professionals about nutrition. She is a Fellow of the American College of Nutrition, a certified nutrition specialist, and a certified functional medicine practitioner. Currently, Dr. Minich teaches for the Institute for Functional Medicine and for the graduate program in human nutrition and functional medicine at the University of Western States. Her passion is bringing forth a whole-self, colorful approach to nourishment and bridging the gaps between science, soul, and art in medicine. Visit her at *www.deannaminich.com*.

TO OUR READERS

Conari Press, an imprint of Red Wheel/Weiser, publishes books on topics ranging from spirituality, personal growth, and relationships to women's issues, parenting, and social issues. Our mission is to publish quality books that will make a difference in people's lives—how we feel about ourselves and how we relate to one another. We value integrity, compassion, and receptivity, both in the books we publish and in the way we do business.

Our readers are our most important resource, and we appreciate your input, suggestions, and ideas about what you would like to see published.

Visit our website at *www.redwheelweiser.com* to learn about our upcoming books and free downloads, and be sure to go to *www.redwheelweiser.com /newsletter* to sign up for newsletters and exclusive offers.

You can also contact us at *info@rwwbooks.com*.

Conari Press
an imprint of Red Wheel/Weiser, LLC
65 Parker Street, Suite 7
Newburyport, MA 01950
www.redwheelweiser.com